# Nutrition and Development

# CURRENT CONCEPTS IN NUTRITION

Myron Winick, Editor

*Institute of Human Nutrition*
*Columbia University College of Physicians and Surgeons*

Volume 1: Nutrition and Development
*Edited by Myron Winick*

# NUTRITION AND DEVELOPMENT

*Edited by*

**MYRON WINICK**

*Institute of Human Nutrition*
*Columbia University College of Physicians and Surgeons*

A WILEY-INTERSCIENCE PUBLICATION,

**JOHN WILEY & SONS,**
New York • London • Sydney • Toronto

**LIBRARY OF CONGRESS CATALOGING IN PUBLICATION DATA**

Winick, Myron.
    Nutrition and development.

    (Current concepts in nutrition, v. 1)
    Includes bibliographies.
    1. Nutrition. 2. Maternal-fetal exchange.
3. Children—Growth. I. Title. II. Series.
[DNLM: 1. Child nutrition—Growth. WS 115 W772n
1972]

RJ131.W55                   612.6′5                72-5097
ISBN 0-471-95440-3
Printed in the United States of America

10 9 8 7 6 5 4 3 2 1

# Preface

This book synthesizes existing knowledge in two areas—nutrition and development—and outlines the important information presently being generated at the interphase of these two disciplines. During the past two decades there has been mounting evidence that the state of nutrition during early life can have a lasting influence on the subsequent development of the organism. While all of the mechanisms involved in this "nutritional programming" are not yet fully understood, certain general principles have been learned. These are dealt with in this book. In addition, some of the biochemical changes induced by early nutrition manipulation are discussed in specific organ systems; mechanisms producing these alterations and explaining their persistence are explored. Finally, these findings are reviewed and examined in terms of their clinical importance and their relevance to the health of children.

In the narrow sense, this book explores the effects of deprivation of specific nutrients on the biochemical development of selected organ systems. It not only details what occurs and how long it lasts but also explores the biochemical mechanisms leading to the observed changes. In the broader sense, however, this book deals with the problem of what we are and how nutrition during our early life may have influenced how we got there.

Myron Winick

*New York, New York*
*April 1972*

# Contents

# Nutrition and Development

# 1

# Development of Physiological Regulations

E. F. ADOLPH

Department of Physiology, The University of Rochester, Rochester, New York

An animal regulates its metabolism. Such a statement is easy to make, but less easy to substantiate. The words "regulates" and "metabolism" are too comprehensive to call up a picture of what happens inside a man or a rat that maintains these vital functions.

Every experimenter in nutrition knows that a growing animal shows effects of changed food intakes and deprivations sooner than an adult animal does. For this reason, among others, we look to "development" for answers to certain questions about metabolism.

These three concepts—regulation, metabolism, and development—often lie unexamined in the minds of bioscientists. By facing some of the phenomena in which they combine we can bring these concepts into the open. That is the purpose of this chapter.

Let me ask two questions and try to answer them. What do active self-regulations mean in the life of an animal, old or young? And, in what steps do particular regulatory arrangements develop in new individuals?

## HEART RATE

The heart beat furnishes an example of physiological regulations at work. An animal's heart beats as fast as it is commanded to beat. What commands it? In bodily rest it maintains an almost minimal rate; that rate depends largely on its intrinsic pacemaker. If the heart is isolated from

This chapter was written with financial support of the National Science Foundation.

the body, it is cut off from most extrinsic influences and in some species maintains nearly the same minimal rate as before isolation. However, it still responds to changes of conditions inside itself, such as mechanical stretch and chemical composition at the pacemaker. But, if the heart remains *in situ*, even the minimal rate also depends on two flows of nerve impulses from the brain's medulla, one flow in the sympathetic system (prodding the heart) and another in the parasympathetic system (restraining it). At heart rates above the minimum the sympathetic flow is usually found to have increased; those nerve impulses are aroused by afferent streams of information coming from many sites of bodily activity. The bodily activities, by this and other means, command increases of blood flow (and oxygen flow) to their sites.

All these influences, intrinsic and extrinsic, are regulating the heart rate. The heart is in part the servant of all tissues that send messages and, in addition, initiates some (reflex) messages itself. Even when most extrinsic influences are cut off, as by complete denervation, the steady rate of beat now adopted still represents regulation. Without intrinsic regulation the heart might behave like a spring-wound toy, running down to zero. Instead, it resembles a self-winding clock. The clock's regulator (pendulum or escapement) ensures that minutes and hours will be uniform in length. The heart's regulator ensures that the pace will be uniform until disturbed and will return to its idling rate after the disturbance has subsided.

When, during the individual's development, does heart rate become regulated? In an embryo the heart's action has a visible beginning; indeed there is no heart in the early embryo. At a certain stage "cardiac" muscle tissue segregates in the embryo's head end (Fig. 1). Hours or

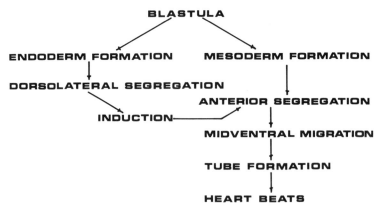

Fig. 1.   Scheme of formative differentiations that precede beating of the heart, based on studies of salamander and chick by various investigators.

days later it starts to contract regularly. Slow at first, the beats increase in frequency throughout much of larval or fetal maturation. Most of the increase of rate during fetal life represents a regulatory change in the pacemaker's norm, a progression in the intrinsic rate. Later, extrinsic factors, one by one, also make themselves felt (Adolph, 5).

Orderly appearance of regulations similar to those governing heart rate is an integral part of all ontogenetic development. By experimental interference with intrinsically programmed events it can be determined when and how the regulatory systems come into action, and, by means to be mentioned, the responses of various systems as they exist at successive stages of partial maturation can be tested.

## WHAT IS REGULATION?

Today's physiologists study chiefly two kinds of phenomenon: (a) processes—what is done in living units and by what means—mechanisms; and (b) regulations—when and how much is done—*quando et quanto*. The two kinds are closely linked in that every process contains not only a conjunction of working parts and materials but also a control of speed and intensity. The study of controls identifies relations among selected activities; namely, those activities that influence speed and intensity. These relations characterize a regulatory arrangement.

Since specific relations are the basis of regulatory arrangements, their study can be considered as belonging in part to a great group of concepts generally termed "field" concepts. Gravitation and electromagnetism belong to this group. Isaac Newton and Clerk Maxwell, who outlined these two studies, respectively, recognized that no one could foreseeably reduce a gravitational field or an electromagnetic field to mechanisms. Therefore we are concerned with a description of "the form of the relation between the motions of the parts" (Maxwell, 34). The probability that isolation of parts would destroy the system under study, that the relations involved are irreducible, has to be faced. Studies of physiological regulations unavoidably include field concepts, for relations between operating parts are being described. Some such relations are illustrated farther on.

Regulation is, then, the automatic self-control over an organism's processes or state. The heart rate shows a resting level and a provision for predictable changes. Protein content or water content of an adult animal's body is about the same, day after day and even year after year, although each is continuously renewed. This sameness indicates that a norm, once established within the body, is maintained through responsive processes (a) of gain or anabolism and (b) of loss or catabolism. Although no one knows what tissue or subcell contains the body's norm or set point for protein or water, the operating characteristics that maintain the norm can be described.

Regulation of a physiological process resembles regulation of a heat system. In a house a designed "regulator," sensitive to the air temperature, turns on and off a switch that activates a heating unit (for gain) or a cooling unit (for loss). Such actions result in a nearly constant temperature at the regulator.

## WHAT IS DEVELOPMENT?

Development of the young individual provides not only new structures and processes but also the tools of physiological regulations. As a zygote changes into an active individual, it (a) *differentiates* or changes qualitatively and (b) *grows* or increases in material and nonmaterial possessions. The quantitative increases are part of the expansion of the numbers of bodily properties.

Differentiation depends on interactions among cells or tissues that have earlier become partially specialized. Thus a heart forms in the mesoderm that happens to lie in contact with endoderm in a particular anterior region of the embryo (Fig. 1). Later, spontaneous contractions arise in a posterior subregion of the tubular cardiac mass; this subregion becomes a pacemaker that determines how frequently the mass will contract.

The interactions among embryonic regions were summarized by Harrison (26):

In regions in which differentiation is not primary but dependent on an organizer or inductor as is the case in the ectoderm of the vertebrate embryo, two fields are involved, the inducing and the induced—each with its intensity gradients, thresholds of activity and sensitivity and each with time limits on its function.

A differentiated region has unique chemical and functional properties as well as unique structures. Without differentiation neither new processes nor new regulations begin to operate.

The aspects of development mentioned here are not those currently emphasized by molecular biologists. They can be scanned elsewhere; for example in Reiner (40, Chapter 6). I speak instead of development in terms of organ activities, which contain molecular elements but exhibit much more than those to the eyes of functional biologists. Each level of description raises problems for those working at higher and lower magnifications; no single description can do justice to them all.

As the developing organism unfolds, visible events appear in an orderly sequence. Each event actually marks a new process or combination of processes. Further, many a process emerges without a visible trigger, appearing "spontaneously." However, it is already controlled in rate by a self-contained pacemaker, the latter term now having the general meaning of a rate controller. Only subsequently is the intrinsic pace of activity modified by extrinsic influences. Such is the once-for-all establishment of each process and each regulatory arrangement.

## TIMING OF DEVELOPMENT

Everyone recognizes that a given characteristic of an individual first appears at a particular age. This age may be regarded as predetermined. The biologist concludes that each structure or process has an onset.

In the study of morphogenesis the biologist ascertains that a structure can be made to appear if at a certain age an inductor acts. He says the tissue has become competent. He finds, by experimentation such as transplantation or hormone administration, that competence prevails only during a specific range of time. A new structure therefore differentiates from mutual effects of competent tissue and potent inductor. The induction determines *what* resultant will emerge (e.g., spontaneous contractions of cardiac fibers). Activation (or triggering) may determine independently *when* the resultant will actually take effect in the normal course of events; for example, when the heart will begin to beat rhythmically.

Similarly, in physiogenesis we observe the appearance of new competence. An illustration is furnished by an experiment of Greengard (24). First, tyrosine aminotransferase (TT) ordinarily appears in rat liver a few hours after birth. Second, TT will appear earlier, a day or two before birth, if either glucagon or epinephrine is injected into the fetus, which shows that TT production is competent to respond to either of these inductors. Third, TT does not appear if the inductor is injected before three days prenatally. Fourth, TT does appear even before three days prenatally if, instead, cyclic AMP is injected. From these tests it may be inferred that glucagon or epinephrine induces formation of cyclic AMP within three days of birth, but not earlier, since the livers of young fetuses are not yet competent to form AMP. But once they become competent they await only the circulation of the hormone to form AMP. Ordinarily the AMP formation is first activated at birth itself.

Another illustration may be cited at the level of organ function. Total arrangements for breathing become competent before birth, as shown by the onset of breathing in premature individuals. The competence awaits activation by issuance of the fetus from the uterus and interruption of blood flow in the umbilical cord.

A specific physiological regulation, then, such as TT production or breathing, is established as a result of developmental interactions and begins to operate when triggered. I next inquire whether a regulation commences all at once or by steps.

## AN EXAMPLE OF REGULATION: WATER CONTENT

First, well-known regulatory arrangements for the adjustment of body water content are described; then the ontogenetic events that lead to their operation are shown.

In an adult dog, for instance, its body's water content depends on two processes, excretion of more water when water is excessive in amount and ingestion of more water when water is deficient in amount (Adolph, 1).

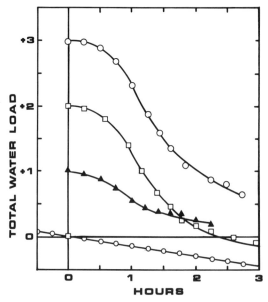

Fig. 2.   Courses of water loads (percent of body weight) during three hours after water (of three amounts) was placed in stomachs of adult dogs. Tolerance curves. From Adolph (1, p. 19).

A typical test of regulation by excretion accordingly consists in place-
ment of a water load in the stomach, followed by periodic measurements
of the amount of load remaining in the body. Elimination of the water
can be measured either by repeated weighings of the animal free of
urine or by collection of the urine as it is produced. For a given water
excess the elimination is gradual over two or three hours (Fig. 2); the
change of body water content constitutes a *water tolerance curve;* simul-
taneous dilution and reconcentration of the blood plasma show a parallel
tolerance curve. For water, as for any other substance in excess, tolerance
of the body is measured by the speed of recovery toward the norm
of body content.

Over a chosen period of time, such as one hour, the rates of water
elimination after various water loads have been given can be compared.
Characteristically, the rates are greater with larger water excesses; the
pertinent graph is a *dose-response curve* (Fig. 3). The "object" of this

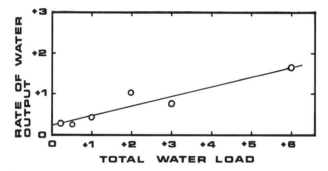

Fig. 3.   Water outputs (percent of body weight in first hour) after administrations
of water by stomach tube (percent of body weight). Adult dogs. Dose-response curve.
From Adolph (1, p. 27).

regulation appears to be the body's water content, and the manner of
regulation resembles that of a proportional regulator.

Next, a typical test of regulation by ingestion consists in the imposition
of various water deficits in dogs by forced evaporation through panting
or by other subtraction of body water. When drinking is thereafter per-
mitted, it cancels the water deficit in a few minutes. Again a proportional
regulator operates to yield another dose-response curve (Fig. 4).

Both activities (elimination and ingestion) represent water *exchanges.*
They tend automatically to maintain that particular bodily *content* of
water at which an hour's eliminatory loss equals an hour's ingestive
gain. The combination of processes ensures a nearly constant content.

An animal has available several pathways of water loss and water

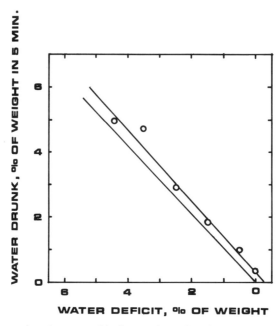

**Fig. 4.** Water intakes (percent of body weight in first five minutes) after water was allowed to adult dogs initially dehydrated to the water deficits (percent of body weight) indicated. Light line represents the hypothesis that intakes equal deficits. Dose-response curve. From Adolph (4, p. 164).

gain, but studies show that loss through only one pathway (renal excretion) increases in response to water excesses and gain through only one pathway (oral ingestion) increases in response to water deficits.

The action of the combined arrangements may be referred to as an *equilibration* of water content, and Fig. 5 is termed an equilibration diagram. Such a diagram includes the results of many tolerance curves, each curve starting from a different administered load.

An important part of regulation is feedback or communication as through a sensory channel, of the extent to which adjustment is progressing. In the case of water content progress of adjustment is partly reflected in the concentration and volume of the excess fluid remaining in the body. *Where* the concentration and the volume are detected is still in some doubt, but one site may be within the brain stem (Verney, 43; Andersson, 10) and another may be within the venous circulation (Gauer and Henry, 22). In general, detectors of the bodily state set up messages that can travel from the detectors to the executive organs.

My answer to the first chief question is now as concrete as present

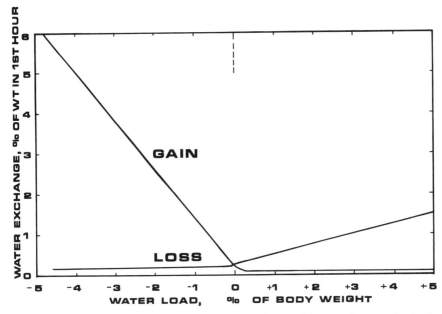

**Fig. 5.** Water exchanges in relation to water loads. Equilibration diagrams for body water in adult dogs. From Adolph (1, p. 32).

understanding can make it: self-regulations are automatic actions that either furnish constancy of cellular or bodily properties or supersede the norms in pursuit of temporary objectives.

## ORIGIN OF WATER EQUILIBRATION

Now comes our account of the development of water regulation. The age of onset of the equilibration arrangement is sought by tests that reveal to what extent newborn dogs respond to water excesses given by stomach. Even though urine be withdrawn periodically from the urinary bladder, little diuresis (increase of water output) is found in a newborn dog loaded with water. This striking result means that the capacity for water diuresis is chiefly acquired some time postnatally. Its onset is actually found 7 to 12 days after birth. Before that age a water load, once administered, remains in the body (Fig. 6), and the blood plasma continues to be diluted during at least three hours.

Similar studies show that not only dog but also man (Ames, 9) and rat (Falk, 19) first activate water diuresis a few days after birth. Yet other agents (epinephrine or hypoxia) can arouse diuresis on the day

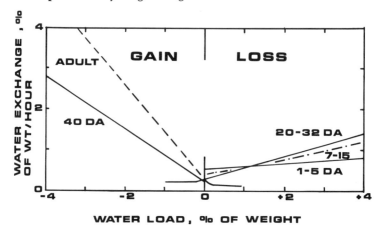

**Fig. 6.** Equilibration diagrams for body water in infant dogs of four ages (*da* = days after birth). From Adolph (5, p. 32).

of birth. Therefore the machinery for varying the urine flow is available, but the response to water excess is small at birth. Further, a stage is found in infant rats at which water diuresis is aroused, but antidiuretic hormone does not inhibit it (Adolph, 2, p. 116). Indeed, in the several species investigated this hormone, though present in the pituitary gland, does not invade the blood until a postnatal age considerably after the capacity for water diuresis is fully established (Krecek and Heller, 30).

What influence may trigger the onset of the capacity for water diuresis is not known. Evidently the trigger is related to the event of birth, for, regardless of the stage of total physiological development at which birth occurs in a given species, water diuresis soon becomes established, and no matter how prematurely an individual may be born water diuresis is promptly acquired (Ames, 9). This fact also illustrates the point that an onset is not wholly keyed to a stereotyped program of development but, like liver TT, may be connected to a movable element of the program such as birth.

Since the ingestion response to water deficit of the body develops after the excretion response to water excess (Fig. 6), it must be concluded that the total pattern of water equilibration materializes in discrete steps.

### EQUILIBRATIONS

How general are arrangements for equilibration of bodily contents and properties? Adjustments by gains and losses have been shown to apply to physiological regulations of (a) body heat and (b) total nutrients. These, like water content, are measurable metabolic states (Adolph, 1, pp. 309 and 327). There are undoubtedly others, and cellular ones, too. The general principle is that for a specific property or component, exchanges of component operate which tend to restore the specific content to its norm or set point. Exchanges of component need not be by intake or output but can result from chemical transformations, local transports, tissue activities, and so on.

Those nutritive substances that interchange in metabolism achieve an internal equilibration by substitution or intermediary transformation. In such instances multiple regulations operate, and the gains and losses are not between body and surroundings but among metabolic pools. In order to measure the load of a single component, the component's volume of distribution and the mean concentration in that volume are measured: their product is the total content. Although the observer of this component is now one stage removed from direct vision of the load and of the exchange, studies to date nevertheless show that water regulation is a model for regulations of nitrogen, amino acids, and glucose. Sodium chloride, at least in sheep and rats, has been found to be specifically ingested in response to deficit (Beilharz et al., 12), a regulation that probably depends on liberation of adrenal corticoids to prompt its ingestion (Fregly, 21). For most other components the intakes and outputs are less specific (Maller, 33), although taste and other qualities serve as partial cues for intake. In general, animals do not detect single components of the various foods they ingest in compensation for deficits; they ingest mixtures.

An equilibration is response to an internal state. Indeed, most responses to internal states serve to regulate some bodily property. Whenever, in an equilibration diagram, the ordinates and the abscissae concern the same component (such as water), a regulatory circuit exists; that is, exchange of $X$ adjusts the content of $X$ itself. Such responses yield homeostasis. The point to be emphasized here is that each such arrangement develops at some stage of ontogeny.

Two levels of regulation can be conveniently distinguished: organismic and cellular. *Organismic* regulations control properties that apply to the whole body and particularly to the fluid medium bathing all tissues. They concern metabolic pools, extracellular volumes and compositions, oxygen supplies, and body temperatures. Special organs effect inputs and outputs and respond to calls for action.

*Cellular* regulations are managed by individual cells. They concern cell compositions and structures, exchanges or transports, rates of chemical transformations, and syntheses of enzymes. Often cell boundaries and organelles furnish sites of response and action. Organismic regulations reduce the number of controls incumbent on individual cells, whereas those regulations that differ from one kind of cell to another necessarily reside in each cell.

Coordinations among regulatory organs, and among cellular organelles, depend on maintained communications. Messages convey mutual influences, as in the case of extrinsic regulations already mentioned.

## MEASUREMENT OF DEVELOPMENT

Growth does not just happen. In each body and tissue it is intrinsically and extrinsically determined. Growth rates, measured by overall increase of bulk, can be experimentally modified in young animals and in specific tissues. Known means of modification are genetic constitutions, nutritive supplies, compensatory hypertrophies after partial excisions, and special factors.

Among the special factors that have been identified are the nerve-growth factor of Levi-Montalcini and Angeletti (31) which promotes multiplication and enlargement of sensory and sympathetic nerve cells; erythropoietin which arouses the excessive formation of erythrocytes; and thyroid hormones which induce metamorphosis in amphibians and hasten maturations in vertebrates generally. In each factor an immediate influence evidently either accelerates or limits the production of tissue, thus demonstrating that ordinary growth is at less than the maximal rate possible.

The fact that growth rates can be influenced does not mean that other developments keep pace with the increase of tissue mass. Indeed, in the above examples single cell types respond more readily than whole tissues or whole bodies. Corresponding to each accelerator of growth, an inhibitor system also operates; both feed information to the regulating and regulated tissue. Thus mitosis of liver cells in adult rats increases in frequency when there is a deficit of plasma proteins and decreases (is inhibited) when there is an excess of plasma proteins (Goss, 23, p. 232). In this case mitosis is a convenient index to the operation of a balanced regulatory system.

In the following paragraphs I describe the courses of development (growth) of several quantitative properties. It is not necessary to know what the regulatory arrangements are to see the results of their actions.

The body's normal water content at various ages can be measured as the fraction of water in the body's total substance, but, since body fat differs among individuals, and especially at various ages, it is customary to record water content as a fraction of fat-free body weight.

Figure 7 shows the courses of water fraction with age from conception (ages on a logarithmic scale) for three species. In all species water

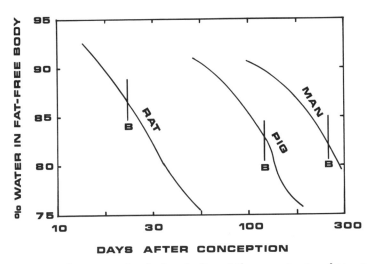

Fig. 7.   Percent of water in the fat-free bodies of three species in relation to age from conception (on logarithmic scale). B = birth. Rat, data of Hohenauer and Oh (27) and Jelinek (28). Pig, data of McCance and Widdowson (35) and Filer and Churella (20). Man, data of Owen et al. (39).

fraction decreases but not uniformly with age. (a) The fastest decreases come at earlier ages in those species with short gestations than in those with long gestations. In fact, the sharpest decrease precedes birth in each species. (b) The rate of decrease is slowest in species with long gestations. To compare among species the velocities of decrease one may estimate how many days it takes for body water to diminish, say, from 90 to 80% of the fat-free tissues. In general, the species with long fetal existence decrease body water not only slowest but also latest.

The decrease of water percentage with age represents chiefly a decrease of extracellular volume in each gram of body. Each tissue becomes tighter as the spaces between cells diminish. Correspondingly, bodily deposition of sodium decreases and potassium increases.

Do the velocity and the timing of maturations also differ among species for other components than water? From among several components for which data are available I choose hemoglobin concentration in blood, arterial blood pressure, and renal clearance of inulin. Although each is measured in different units, each develops with different velocities in the several species.

Thus analytical results show that whereas body content of water changes fastest in rat at about 21 days after conception, which is the time of birth, in pig it changes fastest at about 80 days but before birth (Fig. 7). Hemoglobin concentration in blood increases fastest in rat at 14 days after conception and in pig at about 40 days (Barron et al., 11). Species in which birth is still later in life develop even more slowly and use more of the available time to acquire the same levels of these two components—water and hemoglobin.

In similar fashion arterial blood pressure at rest increases more slowly in species with long gestations than in species with short gestations. To climb from 35 mm mercury pressure to 70 mm it takes a sheep (fetus and infant) five times as long as it takes a rat (Dawes, 16, p. 98).

Inulin clearances per unit of body weight are small at the time of birth and in a few days following birth increase enormously, whether in rat, dog, or sheep (Alexander and Nixon, 8). This component, therefore, awaits birth for its major growth and illustrates the fact that some properties do not synchronize their developments with the development of chemical components of the body as a whole.

Since all development is not maximal at one age, even in one species, I conclude that each property follows a schedule which believedly relates to the rest of growth but in no simple way.

Clearly, two kinds of regulation govern the velocities of formation of a bodily component. (a) The adult kind quickly restores water content, blood pressure, or hemoglobin concentration when either is displaced from the norm. (b) The norm changes with age according to a program; possibly localized RNA messengers determine what the progression will be in body water content, arterial blood pressure, or blood hemoglobin concentration.

## SEQUENCES IN DEVELOPMENT

The ages at which various physiological regulations either begin to act or attain a certain level of action can be compared among species. For this purpose events of physiological development are chosen that happen to be known in a number of mammalian species (Adolph, 7). In this study the events are arbitrarily arranged in the sequential order in which they appear during prenatal and postnatal development of the rat. Ages are represented for convenience on a logarithmic scale (Fig. 8).

Onsets appear, in general, but not always, in the same sequence in

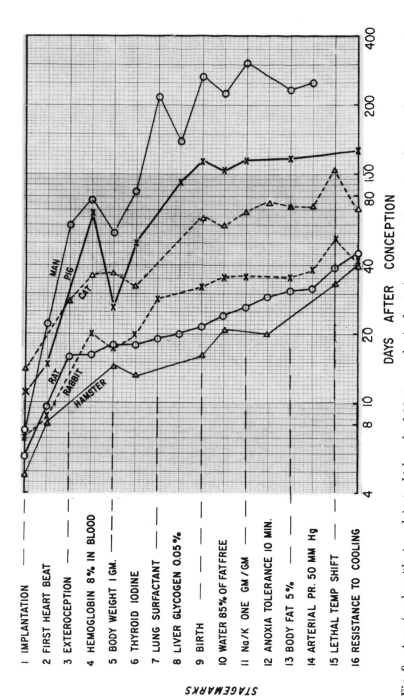

**STAGEMARKS**

1 IMPLANTATION
2 FIRST HEART BEAT
3 EXTEROCEPTION
4 HEMOGLOBIN 8% IN BLOOD
5 BODY WEIGHT 1 GM.
6 THYROID IODINE
7 LUNG SURFACTANT
8 LIVER GLYCOGEN 0.05%
9 BIRTH
10 WATER 85% OF FAT FREE
11 Na/K ONE GM/GM
12 ANOXIA TOLERANCE 10 MIN.
13 BODY FAT 5%
14 ARTERIAL PR. 50 MM Hg
15 LETHAL TEMP SHIFT
16 RESISTANCE TO COOLING

DAYS AFTER CONCEPTION

**Fig. 8.** Ages (on logarithmic scale) at which each of 16 stagemarks (ordinates) appear in six species of mammals, prenatal and postnatal. From Adolph (70), in which sources of data are given.

15

different species; for instance, stagemark #6, the first accumulation of iodine in thyroid gland, appears in some species before stagemark #5, body weight of one gram, in other species after it. There are, therefore, exceptions to the rule that events have a stereotyped sequence in all mammals.

Those species with long gestations ( #9) take longer to develop nearly all stagemarks than do those species with short gestations, as remarked above. Also, stagemarks such as 85% water content ( #10) that appear *after* birth in small species with short gestations appear before birth in large species with long gestations. Hence the events that forerun a particular stagemark in one species are not all required in order to trigger the same stagemark in another species. Evidently more than one sequence or program operates the concurrent timings of development.

Possible interrelations among the onsets of diverse properties can now be visualized; for instance, the rise in arterial blood pressure to 50 mm of mercury ( #14) appears much too late to account for the sudden appearance of water diuresis just after birth in small species. The rise in inulin clearance, however, which, it is usually inferred, equals capsular filtration rate, can be a critical factor in the onset of postnatal water diuresis, for its rise parallels that of water diuresis in several species.

Sequences therefore reveal no simple relation among the onsets of development of various physiological properties, but the map of sequences shows where the problems are that must be solved before development can be viewed as a smooth establishment of one regulation after another.


## COMPOUND DEVELOPMENT

Since physiological properties of an individual are acquired at various ages, the sequential acquisitions taken together add up to an overall development. Moreover, once a property is acquired, it does not remain static; thus, in the case of heart rate, the activity starts under its own pacemaker, and this pacemaker changes with age; eventually it comes under the influence of extrinsic factors, some of which arise in distant organs. In this way rates of activities become modifiable, whether the activities represent chemical syntheses, heart rates, hydrostatic pressures, or nervous impulses. Extrinsic controls tie the rate of a given activity $\alpha$ to other selected activities of the organism and determine what coordinations, priorities, and limits shall exist. Multiple regulation of each property or activity appears to be the rule. This fact can be expressed in a general equation: $R_\alpha = f(A,B,C,$ etc.$)$, which indicates that the resultant of all regulatory influences on $\alpha$ is a function of $A,B,C$, etc., and their interactions. These interactions, often arising separately and serially, communicate with $\alpha$ by mechanical nervous and chemical means, either continuously or intermittently.

## REGULATIONS IN EMBRYO AND FETUS

Specific self-regulations actively maintain the egg and sperm and later the zygote. Thus oxygen is consumed at a fixed rate; permeabilities and active transports equilibrate this component and that. Subsequently new regulated activities emerge; one such is the accumulation of blasto-cyst fluid secreted by trophoblast cells. In rabbit embryos the single-layered cells that surround this fluid push into it a volume of fluid equal to their own cell volume every three minutes (Daniel, 15). Blasto-cyst fluid (extracellular fluid) may be said to manifest almost the earliest physiological regulation exerted by the organism as a whole.

The composition of blastocyst fluid differs significantly from the fluid in the uterine cavity from which it derives—as in concentrations of protein, glucose, and bicarbonate (Lutwak-Mann, 32). At first the pro-teins cannot be distinguished from those of maternal plasma. In later stages new protein constituents of plasma can be recognized as belonging to the fetus and as coming from ribosomes in certain of its liver cells (Wise and Oliver, 45).

Metabolic regulations lend themselves to study at early stages of de-velopment, for a source of nutrients lies available to every embryo. Of these, those substances that pass freely into the embryo could con-ceivably be controlled extrinsically, especially in mammals, but most assimilations or incorporations of materials appear actually to be con-trolled by each fetal organism or specific tissue of it. Water content of an embryonic compartment, as an illustration, is largely determined at boundaries, whether they be body wall, placenta, or cell. At some em-bryonic boundaries permeability to water or to protein is a potent factor of control, but at others fetal water is pumped either directly or indirectly by an active transport (Adolph, 3). The embryo or fetus is therefore not only controlling the number and composition of its cells but also the volume of extracellular fluids and perhaps the pool sizes for most, but not all, components.

Concentrations in plasma appear to be largely self-determined. Some are higher, others lower, in fetus than in mother; for example, plasma chloride and plasma protein are significantly lower in fetuses, but plasma potassium is higher than in adults (Widdowson and McCance, 44). The high potassium concentration of fetal extracellular fluid has been found necessary for the normal differentiation in vitro of the tubular system of fetal mouse kidneys (Crocker and Vernier, 14). On the other hand, the decrease with age in the potassium concentration outside irritable cells is important in increasing the electrical polarization of nerve and muscle fibers, thus making them more excitable (Skoglund, 42). That fetal concentrations are actively regulated follows from the observation that an injection of sodium chloride into the fetal body, increasing the plasma chloride concentration above the maternal, is followed by diminution to a concentration below the maternal (Adolph, 5, p. 35).

As the fetus absorbs nutrients it synthesizes hemoglobin, manufactures specific enzymes, and so on. The rate of each synthesis or other process that can be measured has a control behind it. As mentioned above, these controls supposedly tie every rate to concurrent bodily states.

Cell regulations are especially reflected in the structures and enzymic activities of liver, blood, and other organs of fetuses. Chemical compositions have also been explored to some extent; thus, if the contents of muscle cells (pig, man) in protein nitrogen and in potassium are compared, the ratio N/K is found to increase during prenatal development (Dickerson and Widdowson, 18). This increase suggests that the composition of cells is changing with age, along with the more visible changes in structure.

New activities also appear in fetal organs; the pancreas first forms secretion, the lungs first form surfactant, motor nerves first excite muscles, and synapses first polarize. Each new activity represents a maturation of one property. All are evidence that the fetus controls its own development by instituting regulatory devices for each activity; it does not wait for external stimuli to arouse its first secretions or first movements. The mammalian fetus resembles a bird embryo in its independence; no one supposes that the composition and regulation of a bird are directly controlled by the mother, once the egg has been laid. The bird embryo itself converts the yolk that has been provided into structure and energy of developing tissues; the fetus, however, does not depend on yolk but on inflow of nutrients at the placenta.

That the fetus is, in general, independent of the maternal organism except for supplies is also indicated by the fact that each organ and tissue has its own size and composition at every stage of development. Further, size and composition tend to be independent of changes in maternal composition except when the mother has suffered severe deficiencies or carries an excessive number of fetuses.

The maternal organism is not only source and sink for fetal materials but also furnishes a uniform background or environment of mechanical thermal, and chemical constancy. The fetus is not presented with extremes. Indeed, a few fetal properties, such as body temperature or osmotic pressure of plasma, reflect wholly the regulations contributed by the mother. Hence a profitable distinction can be made between (a) some concentrations that are partly regulated by the mother and (b) the contents of fetal body and organs that are controlled within the fetus. Pools of many components exist in the maternal blood; from them the fetal body "selects," incorporates, and turns over each. In this the fetus and mother divide labor: the maternal body provides digestion, excretion, supply, and constancy; the fetal body furnishes anabolism, catabolism, and growth.

## REGULATIONS IN INFANT

At birth additional regulations start. Some, like enhancement of bilirubin conjugation in liver, are triggered by severance of the placenta. Others, like the control of breathing, are triggered by a complex of sudden events, particularly by the interruption of umbilical blood flow. Other regulations that appear at birth are those reflected in the build-up of blood glucose at the expense of liver glycogen, partly through the agency of newly formed glucose-6-phosphatase, and those activated in the alimentary tract by the first intake of food.

Birth activates more regulatory systems than any other event of a lifetime. Some systems are already in action but shift their set-points, others come out of inhibition, and still others are built anew. Additional regulations appear considerably later than birth, embellishing the bare "necessities" that were ready at birth. Infancy is a period in which self-sufficiencies become more plentiful, and the capacity to respond to variations in environment and in distant organs of the body itself is enhanced.

Tests of regulation that can be applied after birth are those that can be applied to adults.

1. After imposition of a deficit or excess of a specific bodily component or property a gain or loss of that component may be modified (equilibration).

2. After a change of bodily concentrations norms may be restored or recovered (differential maintenance).

3. In extreme circumstances properties may not or may be maintained (homeostasis).

4. Neuromuscular activities may tend to restore properties that have been disturbed (behavioral regulation).

5. Specific processes and organs may be identified as necessary for

the maintenance of steady states or recoveries (tools of regulation).

6. Information from sensors may contribute to maintenance of properties (feedback).

7. Influences may be exerted by one component or regulation on others (extrinsic regulation, integration).

I have now answered the second main question: particular regulatory arrangements are acquired during development according to an inherent program. They are acquired piecemeal at various stages of differentiation and maturation. Each step of acquisition may seem meaningless, but when the last step is complete the flexible management of a particular vital property has been installed for a lifetime.

## OXYGEN UPTAKE

Regulations of two indispensable intakes, oxygen and food, are now discussed more specifically.

Control of oxygen uptake or consumption is unique in that the body has almost no store of oxygen. Basal uptake depends chiefly on factors intrinsic to each tissue, corresponding to the idling speed of the energy transformations. Its pacemaker, presumably, lies in each mitochondrion.

Resting oxygen uptake of a whole organism includes more than that dictated by pacemaker control; particularly, tonus influences and hormonal influences are operating. For the whole body cardiac activity, breathing, visceral actions, and maintenance requiring energy persist. In any form of exercise, however, extrinsic controls predominate over the intrinsic; in every exercised cell the local pacemakers are supplemented and overruled.

Regulation of oxygen uptake in many tissues is limited by factors other than oxygen supply. Fetuses, however, even in the presence of oxygen, may regularly use anaerobic transformations as supplements to the aerobic. In this case other tissues such as maternal liver oxidize the organic acids that form, thus sharing with the fetus the burden of chemical transformations.

Before birth in mammals oxygen comes to the fetus through the placenta. Measurements of the oxygen transfer (blood flow times arteriovenous oxygen difference) have been worked out in fetal sheep (Dawes and Mott, 17; Crenshaw et al., 13); during the last half of gestation the oxygen uptake per unit of fetal mass appears to be constant. After birth it is still unchanged but not for long.

In seven species, including sheep, the oxygen uptake increases sharply in the hours or days following birth (Dawes, 16, p. 194). The uptake is measured at neutrality air temperature for that age and species. If the increases were related to the onset of air breathing, they would probably appear immediately after translation of the individual from aquatic (intrauterine) to terrestrial (postnatal) surroundings. In fact, the increases develop gradually. The mean increase amounts to 35% or more and requires one to seven days to attain its peak, although in rat and man a still longer period may be required. The new environment probably activates the increase in oxygen consumption but not through a recognizable mechanical effect; what kind of shift in controls may be represented has scarcely been surmised.

The capacity for existence without oxygen diminishes in the days following birth. Although immediately after birth 20 to 30 minutes of complete anoxia can be endured by several species (while the body temperature is 37°), after a week the endurance time falls to 5 to 10 minutes (Adolph, 6). At present there is no evidence to show that loss of anaerobic capacity either initiates or necessitates the higher rate of resting aerobic activity.

In subsequent weeks and years of life the resting or basal oxygen uptake per unit of body mass slowly decreases, however body mass be measured. Though mitochondrial enzymic activities, thyroidal hormonal outputs, etc., also decrease moderately throughout life, no one of them is demonstrably a prime controller. In these slow changes with age no regulator appears to be ultimate; regulators may rather be integral parts of reciprocal systems that effect integrations throughout the organism.

## FOOD INTAKE

Intake of food is one means by which the animal body maintains itself in kinetic equilibrium at all postnatal ages. To what extent is nutritive intake determined within the body of a newborn infant and to what extent by extrinsic circumstances?

Most mammals at birth obtain only one food, the one they can suckle from the mother's mammary glands. In instances that have been tested they refuse other foods, although they drink milk from an artificial nipple. How much of the distinction between milk and other liquid foods depends on composition, consistency, and taste and how much on the mechanical and other sensations furnished by the source is largely unknown. Tastes become potent in rats after only a few days of postnatal life. Partial modifications of liquid foods become more acceptable as age increases.

Quantitatively, food intake is regulated to an extent even at the first meal. Newborn dogs whose stomachs have been partly filled with milk through a tube take less milk from the mother than do siblings with empty stomachs (Satinoff and Stanley, 41).

In further stages of development food intake is strictly limited, especially through nervous responses. Litters of suckling rats of various numbers show reproducible limitations; each of a litter of two or three infants receives much more food than each of a litter of 12 or 15 (Kennedy, 29); but the amount taken by two or three is only a fraction of the milk available. Each such infant enlarges its bulk twice as fast but not five times as fast. Some investigators look to immediate factors such as stomach filling for the limitation, others to the processes of assimilation, and others to the infant's storage facilities.

Weaning consists in the search for, and acceptance of, other foods than those obtained by suckling. Usually their acceptance is gradual, suggesting that responses to cues are extensively reorganized and conditioned by trial and error. To what extent error is recognized is a vital problem. Parental and sibling example determines some acceptances. Infants of all ages, at least in rats, depend to greater extents than adults do on frequent and regular intakes.

Tests of intake control may therefore be applied at various ages. They are amount of food accepted, number of infants supplied by one mother, intake response to previous inanition, artificial weaning, dilution of food by roughage or water, composition of food, response to cold environment, response to bodily dehydration, parenteral feeding, stomach loading, and hypothalamic lesions. In each such experimental situation adjustments of intake or of bodily activity are revealed; each reflects part of a built-in regulatory system consisting largely of nervous elements.

Rats, at least, do not always distinguish a food mixture adequate for survival from one that leads to death even while the adequate mixture is available (Harper, 25). Capacities to distinguish among foods have an ontogeny about which there is much to be learned. Foods that fulfill an internal satisfaction or well-being do so during and after an ontogeny of which the constituent factors are unknown.

## INFANT STORES AND TURNOVERS

Of particular interest are the unique arrangements by which infants retain metabolic excesses that adults would excrete. The arrangements are tested by forced administrations of measured excesses of nitrogen, potassium, phosphorus, or chloride (McCance and Widdowson, 37). The newborn rat or pig retains most of the excess, much as it retains water excess. The view that the means of elimination are simply inadequate fails to recognize that the infant utilizes the excess eventually. The newborn individual is regularly acquiring other bodily constituents and laying down the set proportions of them in tissues. So rapidly is tissue laid down in pig or dog that 90% of the nitrogen in forced excess, as well as in ordinary intake, is retained (McCance and Widdowson, 36).

Apparently expansion of pool size is a partial alternative to excretion. Available pool sizes in the growing animal are clearly much larger per unit of mass than in the adult animal. For some components this pool size relates to the fact that extracellular fluid volume is relatively large in infants.

Constancy of bodily composition and change of bodily composition both imply a continual *turnover* of each bodily component, even in fetus or infant, for no constituent remains in cell or body forever; some is lost and replaced daily, whether it be inorganic ion or protein enzyme. Turnover of most ingesta is ordinarily at constant rate; that rate evidently has a pacemaker governing the catabolism, the anabolism, or both. The constitution of a pacemaker in specific instances cannot be stated, but wherever enzymes are involved their activities or their substrates are probably concerned. Thus tryptophan peroxidase suddenly appears at birth in the liver of rabbit, rises to a fixed value, and remains there (Nemeth, 38). Here it is inferred, as usual, that tryptophan is decomposed at rates depending on the amount of enzyme and on the amount of tryptophan present in liver cells, but both quantities in turn are controlled by some further arrangement: enzyme presumably through RNA composition and tryptophan through proteolysis. In their turn these two processes are also regulated; their means of regulation await further investigation.

## SUMMARY

This chapter describes in a provisional way some of the onsets of physiological regulations that have been partly explored. Each example cited will contribute eventually to a systematic concept of how growth and development achieve a self-sufficient adulthood.

Clearly, development follows a program, most of which is present in a latent form within the zygote. Present views emphasize that arrangements of DNA in differentiating cells dictate such programs. The DNA at one time and place is believed to activate specific RNAs, which determine what enzymes will be synthesized. Remarkable features of development are the stereotyped sequences and concordant timing of the differentiations which activate the onset of physiological regulations.

Each regulation depends on specific responses, some of which appear to develop independently of others. When they materialize, they work, in conjunction with arrangements already present, to form a regulatory system that lasts a lifetime.

At every stage the environment influences development. In early embryos cells adapt to their neighboring cells. In mammals this sort of influence is revealed to a restricted extent by transplantation or culture of zygotes or blastocysts. In other animals the whole development can be modified by experimentally diverse external circumstances. Evidently embryos are sensitive not only to temperature and oxygen pressure but to specific maternal proteins, hormones, and electrolytes.

Regulations present in the developing individual are therefore both those that typically operate intrinsically and those that are imposed from other tissues of the same individual. The total pattern of regulations constitutes a complex of influences which the biologist can reduce to single factors only in part. Rather he is led to recognize the remarkable control exerted by the combined conditions for maintenance—the "field" system. This operating control is presumably provided by a heredity that has been refined by natural selection.

## REFERENCES

1. E. F. Adolph, *Physiological Regulations.* New York: Ronald, 1943, 502 pp.
2. E. F. Adolph, *Quart. Rev. Biol.* **32**: 89–137 (1957).
3. E. F. Adolph, *Quart. Rev. Biol.* **42**: 1–39 (1967).
4. E. F. Adolph, *Handb. Physiol., Amer. Physiol. Soc.* **6**, i, 163–171 (1967).
5. E. F. Adolph, *Origins of Physiological Regulations.* New York, Academic, 1968, 147 pp.
6. E. F. Adolph, *Respir. Physiol.* **7**: 356–368 (1969).
7. E. F. Adolph, *Growth* **34**: 114–124 (1970).
8. D. P. Alexander and D. A. Nixon, *Nature* **194**: 483–484 (1962).
9. R. G. Ames, *Pediat.* **12**: 272–282 (1953).
10. B. Andersson, *Acta Physiol. Scand.* **28**: 188–201 (1953).
11. D. H. Barron et al., Blood and Other Body Fluids. *Biol. Handb., Fed. Am. Soc. Exptl. Biol.*, 114–115 (1961).
12. S. Beilharz, D. A. Denton, and J. R. Sabine, *J. Physiol.* (*London*) **163**: 378–390 (1962).

13. C. Crenshaw, W. E. Huckabee, L. B. Curet, L. Mann, and D. H. Barron, *Quart. J. Exptl. Physiol.* **53**: 65–75 (1968).
14. J. F. S. Crocker and R. L. Vernier, *Science* **169**: 485–487 (1970).
15. J. C. Daniel, Jr., *Amer. Naturalist* **98**: 85–98 (1964).
16. G. S. Dawes, *Foetal and Neonatal Physiology*. Chicago, Yearbook, 1968, 247 pp.
17. G. S. Dawes and J. C. Mott, *J. Physiol. (London)* **146**: 295–315 (1959).
18. J. W. T. Dickerson and E. M. Widdowson, *Biochem. J.* **74**: 247–257 (1960).
19. G. Falk, *Amer. J. Physiol.* **181**: 157–170 (1955).
20. L. J. Filer and H. Churella, *Ann. N.Y. Acad. Sci.* **110**: 380–394 (1963).
21. M. J. Fregly in *The Chemical Senses and Nutrition*, M. R. Kare and O. Maller, Eds. Baltimore, Johns Hopkins, 1967, 115–138.
22. O. Gauer and J. P. Henry, *Klin. Wochensch.* **34**: 356–366 (1956).
23. R. J. Goss, *Adaptive Growth*. New York: Academic, 1964, 360 pp.
24. O. Greengard, *Science* **163**: 891–895 (1969).
25. A. E. Harper in *The Chemical Senses and Nutrition*, M. R. Kare and O. Maller, Eds. Baltimore: Johns Hopkins, 1967, 155–167.
26. Harrison, R. G., 1969. *Organization and Development of the Embryo*. New Haven: Yale, 1969, p. 260, 290 pp.
27. L. Hohenauer and W. Oh, *J. Nutr.* **99**: 23–26 (1969).
28. J. Jelinek, *Physiol. Bohemoslov.* **10**: 249–266 (1961).
29. G. C. Kennedy, *Handb. Physiol., Amer. Physiol. Soc.* **6**, i, 337–351 (1967).
30. J. Krecek and J. Heller, *Proc. XXII Internat. Congr. Physiol.* **1**: 53–59 (1962).
31. R. Levi-Montalcini and P. U. Angeletti, *Quart. Rev. Biol.* **36**: 99–108 (1961).
32. C. Lutwak-Mann, *Nature* **193**: 653–654 (1962).
33. O. Maller in *The Chemical Senses and Nutrition*. M. R. Kare and O. Maller, Eds. Baltimore: Johns Hopkins, 1967, 201–212.
34. J. C. Maxwell, 1865. *Phil. Trans. Roy. Soc. (London)* **155**: 459–512 (1865).
35. R. A. McCance and E. M. Widdowson, *Quart. J. Exp. Physiol.* **41**: 1–17 (1956).
36. R. A. McCance and E. M. Widdowson, *J. Physiol. (London)* **133**: 373–384 (1956).
37. R. A. McCance and E. M. Widdowson, *J. Physiol., (London)* **141**: 81–87 (1958).
38. A. M. Nemeth, *J. Biol. Chem.* **234**: 2921–2924 (1959).
39. G. M. Owen and J. Brozek, in Human Development F. Falkner, Ed. Philadelphia: Saunders, 1966. 644 pp.
40. J. M. Reiner, in The Organism as an Adaptive Control System. Englewood Cliffs, New Jersey: Prentice-Hall, 224 pp, 1968. Chapter 6.
41. E. Satinoff and W. C. Stanley, *J. Compar. Physiol. Psychol.* **56**: 66–68 (1963).
42. S. Skoglund, *Acta Societ. Med. Upsal.* **72**: 76–84 (1967).
43. E. B. Verney, *Proc. Roy. Soc. (London)* **135B**: 25–106 (1947).
44. E. M. Widdowson and R. A. McCance, *Clin. Sci.* **15**: 361–365 (1956).
45. R. W. Wise and I. T. Oliver, *Biochem. J.* **100**: 330–333 (1966).

# 2

# Enzyme Development and Nutrition

IVAN T. OLIVER and DESMOND YEUNG

Department of Biochemistry, University of Western Australia

Innumerable studies have been made on the changes in the activities of tissue enzymes which follow dietary manipulation of experimental animals. Although such studies yield specific information about particular protein species, it seems unlikely that the general descriptive phenomena will differ in substance from those revealed by studies of overall protein synthesis in the experimental dietary situation. Miller (38) has already extensively reviewed the latter area, and it seems premature, therefore, to offer a review that can only elaborate in a more detailed fashion the modulation of the levels of specific proteins that can be brought about by dietary change. In addition, attempts to integrate the descriptive phenomena have not yet yielded particularly lucid theories of tissue mechanisms for dietary effects.

The mechanisms by which preexisting enzyme levels are modulated in adult differentiated tissues almost certainly differ from those that operate in the initial production of a particular enzyme by a differentiating cell, and in considering enzyme development and nutrition we propose to restrict discussion to the latter area. For the purposes of this review enzyme development is defined as the *initial* induction of specific enzyme synthesis. Induction has often been used to describe the stimulation of the rate of enzyme synthesis in situations in which specific enzyme synthesis is already in progress, as in adult differentiated tissues. Satisfactory operational criteria for initial induction would be the appearance of specific enzyme activity or proenzyme in tissues not previously possessed of such specific protein. This situation implies *de novo* synthesis of the unique protein. Attention is concentrated on the effects of a dietary restriction or supplementation on the initial induction of enzymes. An attempt at a critical appraisal of the problems is made and guidelines for future experimental work are suggested.


## ENZYME DEVELOPMENT IN MAMMALIAN TISSUES

The current resurgence of interest in chemical embryology or developmental biochemistry has been stimulated to some extent by pediatric problems related to the management of genetic errors in metabolism, many of which are not clinically apparent until after the birth of the fetus. The newborn infant animal must make rapid readjustment to the new environment which involves respiration, alimentation, and the metabolic ability to utilize new dietary components, and such readjustments turn out to involve in many instances the *de novo* production of previously undetectable enzyme systems. Much descriptive information is now available regarding neonatal enzyme development in various tissues. Experiments to elucidate the mechanisms of the initial induction of such enzyme systems have been stimulated by work on hormonal effects on enzyme synthesis in adult animals (e.g., Lin and Knox, 35), and the theories of gene control in the inducible enzyme systems in bacteria have provided a plausible model to direct more recent work (Jacob and Monod, 27). Accordingly, agents that block DNA-directed RNA synthesis or abort or inhibit protein synthesis have been shown to block the production of a large number (if not all) of the enzymes that first appear in the neonatal period of life, and the evidence continues to accumulate that such processes represent the activation or derepression of previously inactive genes.

Recent work on the effects of nutritional deprivation during pregnancy and neonatal life has revealed that nutritional factors play an important role in determining patterns of protein synthesis and limits of cell division in the young animal (see Miller, 38, for review), but their role in *de novo* synthesis of specific enzymes has not been intensively investigated. It is clear that inadequate dietary provision of essential amino acids will have an effect on the rate of synthesis of apoenzymes or proenzymes, and it is similarly clear that holoenzyme activity will be affected by deprivation of certain vitamins whose metabolic derivatives function as coenzymes or prosthetic groups. Some claims have also been made for the specific induction of enzymes in mammalian tissues by their specific substrates, and such hypotheses clearly draw their inspiration from the inducible systems in bacteria. The contemporary evidence for substrate induction of enzymes is examined first.

ENZYME "INDUCTION" BY SPECIFIC SUBSTRATES

Tryptophan Oxygenase (Pyrrolase) (EC 1.13.1.12)

This enzyme catalyses the conversion of tryptophan to formylkynurenine and exists in the rat essentially only in the liver. It initiates the intermediary metabolism of the amino acid. It has been known for some time that the activity of the enzyme is increased by the administration of tryptophan to adult animals (Knox and Auerbach, 33; Goldstein, Stella, and Knox, 15; Greengard and Feigelson, 20). Increases in the stead-state level of an enzyme activity, however, can be due to either an increase in its rate of synthesis or a decrease in its rate of degradation. The tryptophan "induction" was insensitive to actinomycin D (Greengard and Feigelson, 21), and the enzyme appeared to have a very rapid rate of turnover in vivo (Feigelson, Dashman, and Margolis, 13). For these reasons the situation was reexamined by Schimke and his colleagues and the data and conclusions have been reviewed by Schimke (47). Tryptophan oxygenase of rat liver was purified to immunological purity and an antiserum was obtained. This allowed the precipitation of the enzyme protein from liver extracts. Pulse labeling experiments with $^{14}$C-leucine followed by isolation of the labeled enzyme protein showed that the rate of enzyme synthesis was increased about fivefold during induction with hydrocortisone but was unchanged by tryptophan administration, even though the enzyme activity increased considerably. In a further series of experiments the enzyme was prelabeled with $^{14}$C-leucine in control (uninduced) animals, and it was shown that the amount of labeled enzyme continually diminished thereafter, even though no change in the level of activity occurred. By contrast, when tryptophan was administered, the enzyme activity increased, but there was no decrease in the amount of prelabeled enzyme over nine hours. Thus the conclusion was reached that the rate of synthesis of tryptophan oxygenase is increased by hydrocortisone but that tryptophan prevents enzyme degradation with no effect on the rate of synthesis. A further effect of tryptophan is the activation of the apoenzyme by stimulation of its combination with the haematin prosthetic group (Greengard and Feigelson, 20). Thus in the apparent "induction" by tryptophan accumulation of enzyme occurs as a result of stabilization by the substrate in the presence of continued enzyme synthesis.

Tryptophan oxygenase activity is absent from the fetal rat, rabbit, and guinea pig liver and appears for the first time in postnatal life (see Kretchmer, Greenberg, and Sereni, 34, for a bibliography). Premature delivery of fetuses by uterine section brings about the precocious appearance of enzyme activity (Nemeth, 40, 41). The mechanism of induction of the enzyme in neonatal animals is by no means clear, but the relevant data has been extensively reviewed by Greengard (17). Postnatal development of activity is not prevented by actinomycin D or by adrenalectomy, even though hydrocortisone has been shown to stimulate the rate of synthesis of the enzyme in the adult (Schimke, 47). Tryptophan promotes the conversion of apoenzyme to the haematin containing holoenzyme and in the presence of ascorbate to the active (reduced) holoenzyme (Knox, 32), but in the early stages of the post-natal appearance of activity the enzyme in rat liver is entirely in the holoenzyme form. According to the data of Nemeth (40), tryptophan administration to postnatal rats has only marginal effects on the development of activity, a result to be expected from the fact that the enzyme is almost entirely in the holoenzyme form. The results of experiments with actinomycin D strongly suggest that some unidentified inductive event takes place well before the appearance of active enzyme. This initial event is presumably gene transcription, but it could also be followed by accumulation of apoenzyme, so that a later activation mechanism operates to produce active enzyme. It should be possible to test this hypothesis by using an immunochemical technique to detect apoenzyme. Such a situation has already been suggested by the results of Pitot and Cho (43) who claimed that a protein fraction from adult rat liver promoted activation of tryptophan oxygenase when incubated with fetal-liver microsomes. The factor appeared to be absent from fetal liver. Thus still another event in postnatal appearance of enzyme activity might be the induction of synthesis of such a required protein factor. Several pertinent questions remain to be answered in this system:

1. When does gene transcription occur in relation to the time of appearance of active enzyme?

2. Is gene transcription followed by translation to apoenzyme or does it occur closer to the appearance of activity?

3. If apoenzyme preexists for some time before activation, what is its turnover rate?

4. What is the role of the protein fraction described in adult liver by Pitot and Cho?

All these questions could doubtless be answered by using contemporary methodology. Further work is obviously needed on this system but the weight of the evidence to date suggests that tryptophan is not involved in the initial induction of liver tryptophan oxygenase and the physiological signals remain to be discovered.

## Tyrosine α-Ketoglutorate Aminotransferase (EC 2.6.1.5)

Tyrosine metabolism is multidirectional in mammalian tissues, but the first step on the homogentisate pathway is transamination to p-hydroxyphenyl pyruvate catalyzed by tyrosine aminotransferase. This enzyme is in highest activity in the liver. The pioneer work in Knox's labortatory on the stimulation of enzyme activity by hydrocortisone in adult rats has led to an avalanche of studies on this system over the last few years. The original paper by Lin and Knox (35) showed that the administration of either tyrosine or hydrocortisone led to large increases in hepatic tyrosine aminotransferase activity. In these early studies, however, it was already apparent that the "inductive" effect of substrate was evocable only in the presence of glucocorticoids, since adrenalectomy abolished the effect, and tyrosine "induction" in such animals was achieved only when small doses of hydrocortisone were simultaneously administered.

Kenney and Flora (31) later showed that similar inductive effects could be obtained in intact animals with tryptophan, celite, and bentonite and attributed the activity of such compounds to a "stress" effect that resulted in the release of adrenal cortical hormones, since all the agents were ineffective in adrenalectomized animals. They also showed that all the agents potentiated the inductive effect of small doses of hydrocortisone in adrenalectomized animals. Methionine was active in these experiments but inactive in intact rats, an effect that remains unexplained.

In a later paper Kenney and Albritton (30) verified an earlier suspicion (Kenney and Flora, 31) that tyrosine or celite administration depressed the transaminase level when administered to adrenalectomized animals (see also Rosen and Milholland, 45). They suggested that these effects were due to unspecific stress. In a footnote to the earlier paper it was also reported that tyrosine administration to newborn rats is without effect on the postnatal development of enzyme activity.

Tyrosine aminotransferase is effectively absent from fetal rat liver and develops activity within a few hours of birth (Sereni, Kenney, and Kretchmer, 48). Activity can be precociously induced by premature delivery by uterine section in the rabbit (Litwack and Nemeth, 36), in the rat (Holt and Oliver, 23), and in the mouse (Chuah and Oliver, unpublished experiments). In rats delivered by uterine section the injection of tyrosine or tryptophan at delivery gives only marginal effects on the subsequent development of activity (Holt and Oliver, unpublished experiments); tyrosine thus appears to play no essential role in the initial induction of tyrosine aminotransferase.

## Liver Glucokinase (EC 2.7.1.2)

Glucokinase is an enzyme found in mammalian tissues which catalyses the phosphorylation of glucose by ATP. The enzyme is characterized by a low affinity for glucose (Dipietro, Sharma, and Weinhouse, 8) and is found in the liver. The enzyme is undoubtedly the rate-limiting step for overall utilization of glucose by the adult liver. In the adult rat it was claimed by Niemeyer, Clark-Turri, and Rabajille (42) that glucose induced enzyme activity. This interpretation was based on the results of glucose-refeeding experiments after fasting and the administration of high fat diets. The best argument against glucose induction was the finding of very low glucokinase activities in the liver of alloxan-diabetic rats, which, of course, have high blood glucose levels (Dipietro and Weinhouse, 9), and the subsequent demonstration of the necessity for insulin in the resynthesis of glucokinase in alloxan-diabetic rats (Salas, Vinuela, and Sols, 46; Sharma, Manjeshwar, and Weinhouse, 49).

The initial development of glucokinase activity was shown to occur during postnatal life by Walker (56) and Ballard and Oliver (3). In the rat the enzyme first appears at about the fifteenth or sixteenth postnatal day. Walker and Holland (57) made an extensive study of factors that might influence the initial production of the enzyme. Results of experiments with amino acid analogs, puromycin, and actinomycin D, all of which prevent the accumulation of enzyme activity in the liver during the developmental phase, are consistent with the notion of initial induction of the enzyme; that is, the enzyme appears to be synthesized *de novo* following gene transcription and translation processes. Attempts to induce enzyme activity before the sixteenth postnatal day by administration of glucose, insulin, or both agents were conspicuously unsuccessful. There was a slight effect of daily glucose injections at the fourteenth day but no effect between 3 and 12 days postnatal. At the time of normal appearance of the enzyme, however, the system responded to stimuli that are effective in the adult animal; that is, starvation reduced the subsequent development of activity and alloxan administration also prevented subsequent enzyme accumulation. In starved animals the enzyme level responded to refeeding with glucose and in the alloxan-diabetic to insulin administration. This data also demonstrates a requirement for insulin in the postnatal initial synthesis of glucokinase and yields no evidence for substrate induction by glucose, since the blood glucose levels of postnatal rats after the first few postnatal hours are normal and daily injections of glucose fail to preinduce the enzyme.

The inductive mechanism for this enzyme thus remains unknown, but the data of Walker and Holland (57) strongly suggest that the neonatal liver develops a capacity to respond to insulin in this specific way on or about day 16. There appears to be no information regarding either the nature of such a response or the nature of the signals that set up the response.

In summary it might be said that there is effectively no evidence of substrate induction of liver glucokinase by glucose either in the adult animal or as part of the mechanism of its initial induction in the neonatal animal.

In this section of the review we have not attempted an exhaustive survey of the literature pertaining to claims of substrate induction in mammalian tissues but have chosen those few cases in which some attempt has been made to determine the role of substrate in the initial induction of enzyme; in other words the role of substrate in enzyme development, as we have defined it, has been examined.

## ENZYME "INDUCTION" BY COFACTORS

Since many vitamins are metabolically converted into cofactors and prosthetic groups of enzymes, it is obvious that dietary deprivation should lead to a reduction in the activities of enzymes that require such cofactors. There will obviously be differential effects among different enzymes, since affinity constants of enzymes for the same cofactor are different. It is not the prime purpose of this section to examine the variation in preexisting enzyme activities following cofactor (or precursor) deprivation but rather to examine the evidence of specific cofactor effects on the initial induction of the apoenzyme molecule.

Unfortunately there appear to be few studies that bear directly on this problem mainly because most experiments on cofactor effects have been performed in adult animals. However, we discuss a few of the studies made in neonatal animals that approach the objectives of this review.

Stimulation of specific apoprotein synthesis by the prosthetic group of the conjugated protein has been reported to occur in hemoglobin synthesis in the reticulocyte (Grayzel, Horchner, and London, 16), but the heme prosthetic group does not seem to be implicated in the initiation of globin synthesis. A few isolated studies of the effects of pyridoxine on specific enzyme synthesis may serve to point up the problems of both experimentation and interpretation in this area.

## Pyridoxine Deficiency and L-Amino Acid Decarboxylase (EC 4.1.28)

Eberle and Eiduson (12) chose to study the enzyme 5-hydroxy-tryptophan decarboxylase in postnatal brain and liver. Earlier studies had shown that pyridoxine deficiency in weanling rats markedly depressed the decarboxylase activity in the liver but had little effect on the brain enzyme (Davis, 7; Wiss and Weber, 58). In the 1968 study the authors examined the effects of pyridoxine deficiency on 5-hydroxy-tryptophan decarboxylase activity in the brains and livers of young rats from mothers to which pyridoxine-deficient diets had been administered for the whole period of two weeks before mating through 16 days after parturition. The authors made measurements of holoenzyme activity by assay of the enzyme in the absence of its added cofactor, pyridoxal phosphate, and of "maximal" enzyme by assay in the presence of saturating concentrations of the cofactor. The growth of both control and deficient fetal rats was the same, as were the growth rates of the organs studied. Differences in growth rates appeared only in the postnatal rats.

Decarboxylase activities were determined in liver, cerebellum, cerebal cortex, and the brain "remainder." The enzyme activities in the liver of newborn rats were effectively the same in both control and deficient groups, and in the control group the maximal and holoenzyme activity increased three- to fourfold over the first 16 days postpartum. In the deficient group, as might be expected, due to cofactor deprivation, the holoenzyme activity fell over this period to about one-third of the activity found in the newborn; the "maximal" enzyme, which is a measure of apoenzyme plus holoenzyme, also showed a slight fall compared with the threefold rise in the control animals. The difference in enzyme activity between control and deficient animals at the sixteenth postnatal day was significant ($P \leq 0.01$). Essentially similar data were obtained in the cortex, cerebellum, and brain remainder, except that there appeared to be some "sparing" of the brain enzyme, since a falloff in maximal enzyme activity was scarcely apparent in the deficient animals.

No evidence of the presence of inhibitors in deficient rat tissues or of activators in nondeficient rat tissues was found by the usual mixing experiments. It is unfortunate that in this study enzyme activities were not determined during the gestation period, since the tissues examined, with perhaps one exception, appear to have initiated enzyme synthesis *in utero*. Activities in the cortex, brain remainder, and liver were all readily detectable in newborn animals, although the authors' use of animal groups 0 to 4 days old may have hidden some valuable information. In the cerebellum of newborn animals the total enzyme activity on a wet-weight basis was similar to that found in the cortex, despite the authors' statement that the enzyme normally appears in measurable activity only during the second week of life. The activity in both cortex and cerebellum was only 10% of the liver activity and 2% of that found in the brain remainder. The holoenzyme activity in the cerebellum and cortex of deficient animals was close to the lower limits of detection.

The study appears to show that pyridoxine deprivation throughout gestation has no effect on the initial induction of 5-hydroxytryptophan decarboxylase in any of the tissues studied, although there is no information about the timing of the event and the enzyme may be constitutive in mammalian organisms. There is clear evidence during postnatal deprivation of pyridoxine that there is a failure in both brain and liver to accumulate the enzyme apoprotein as measured by the maximal enzyme activity. It is important to emphasize that the measurement of maximal enzyme activity is the important parameter here, since it is directly related to the amount of enzyme protein. The holoenzyme content of the tissue is not a direct measure of enzyme protein, since it depends on both the amount of apoenzyme and the amount of cofactor available. Similarly, although it is of interest to measure the holoenzyme, total enzyme protein ratio, and thus the percentage saturation of apoenzyme with cofactor, it is not particularly informative to calculate the absolute amount of apoenzyme (maximal minus holoenzyme), since this figure is only a number whose biological significance is doubtful. Pyridoxine deficiency thus appears to restrict the postnatal accumulation of total decarboxylase protein in rat tissues, but there is no available evidence to show whether the effect is due to the inhibition of apoenzyme synthesis or to the stimulation of enzyme degradation. The operation of either mechanism (or both) could account for the results.

## Tyrosine Aminotransferase (EC 2.6.1.5)

Injections of pyridoxine in adult animals at a dose rate of 60 mg/100 g body weight have been shown to elevate tyrosine aminotransferase activity in the liver (Holten, Wicks, and Kenney, 26). The mechanism of this effect is not clear, but since the enzyme is usually assayed under conditions of saturation with its cofactor, pyridoxal phosphate, the increase in activity almost certainly reflects an increase in the steady-state concentration of apoenzyme protein. It is not unlikely that such an increase is due to stress-potentiated release of adrenal steroids, but recent data of Holt and Oliver (24, 25) suggest a more specific action.

Tyrosine aminotransferase activity first appears in rat liver within a few hours of birth (see p. 31). Holt and Oliver (24) reported the effect of pyridoxine injections in neonatal animals on the subsequent development of enzyme activity. At a dose rate of 60 mg/100 g body weight the injection of pyridoxine into rat fetuses 12 hours before their delivery by uterine section resulted in approximately 50% reduction in the enzyme activity that subsequently developed in saline-injected littermate controls. When pyridoxine was injected at delivery, the repressive effect was lessened but still apparent.

On the other hand, the injection of pyridoxine in two-day postnatal rats, when the enzyme activity has fallen to basal level, resulted in large increases (twofold to sevenfold) in tyrosine aminotransferase activity. In subsequent work Holt and Oliver (25) reported the occurrence of three anionic forms of tyrosine aminotransferase in rat liver which were separable by electrophoresis in polyacrylamide gel. Each form appears to be specifically under discrete hormonal control and the least anionic form is produced after pyridoxine injection in two-day postnatal rats. This form is also produced after insulin injection but is not evoked by hydrocortisone, glucagon, adrenalin, or 3′,5′-cyclic adenosine monophosphate, the other agents implicated in the inductive mechanisms for this enzyme. Thus even the massive doses of pyridoxine do not appear to produce their effect through release of adrenal steroids. The reasons for these opposite effects of pyridoxine in newborn and postnatal rats are not yet known, but there is no good experimental evidence to implicate pyridoxine in the initial induction of tyrosine aminotransferase in the newborn animal. The high doses used may have toxic or pharmacological effects and thus produce repression. In addition, the pyridoxine (and insulin)-induced form of the enzyme does not make its appearance in the liver of neonatal animals until about three days after parturition (Holt and Oliver, 25a). This system, however, is ideally suited to an experimental assessment of the effect of cofactor deprivation on the initial induction of a liver enzyme.

1. The enzyme occurs in three forms, but the precise form stimulated by pyridoxine can be identified.

2. It has been shown by several authors that postnatal development of the enzyme activity is a resultant of *de novo* synthesis (for bibliography see Holt and Oliver, 23, 24).

3. The system has multiple forms of an enzyme catalyzing a single reaction, presumably sharing the same cofactor, but demonstrating a complexity of individual control mechanisms on the induction of each form. For this reason studies of interactions within a complex protein synthetic system resulting from dietary manipulation might well be made.

## POSTNATAL DIETARY CHANGES AND ENZYME DEVELOPMENT

Most of the work reviewed in this section would more properly be discussed under a heading of adaptive changes in enzyme levels in response to dietary changes in young animals. In most instances the effects of weaning to diets of differing constitution and preweaning to synthetic diets in young animals have been monitored by following the changes in preexisting enzyme levels. In some cases, however, the apparent change in the steady-state level of an enzyme may in fact be due to the initial induction of a previously absent isozyme. Such cases deserve closer attention, since they may turn out to be proper subjects for review in future discussions of enzyme development and nutrition. In other cases that fulfill the criteria defined for initial induction it is shown that dietary factors appear to operate through a series of physiological signals, starting at the hormonal level and culminating at intracellular small molecule effectors for inductive events. Most of the work to be reviewed has been on liver enzyme systems because the patterns of postnatal and prenatal induction of enzymes in this tissue has been most extensively charted in recent years. Some of the work to be discussed points up problems of methodology about which some experimental action can now be taken.

### Galactokinase (EC 2.7.1.6)

The capacity of mammalian liver to phosphorylate galactose is due to the specific enzyme galactokinase. Ballard and Oliver (3) showed that the in vitro capacity of rat liver to incorporate $^{14}C$ from galactose into glycogen developed in late fetal life, reached a maximum at about 10 days postnatal, and then fell off toward an adult value of about one-fifth the postnatal maximum. This study was an indirect measure of galactose phosphorylation, but Cuatrecasas and Segal (6) subsequently confirmed the finding by direct measurement of galactokinase activity. The developmental pattern was similar to that obtained by Ballard and Oliver.

Cuatrecasas and Segal suggested that a fetal and adult form of galactokinase might exist, since they found some differences in both kinetic and inhibitory parameters in crude enzyme preparations from each tissue. However, the evidence is not particularly convincing and the postnatal developmental pattern does not suggest replacement of one preexisting enzyme by a new form. These authors also made an attempt to assess the effect of galactose on the developmental pattern of the enzyme. Feeding galactose at the level of 40% of the diet to rats at 16, 18, and 24 days postnatal brought about slight retardation in the decline of enzyme activity which normally occurs over this period. Withdrawal of galactose from the diet at day 16 caused galactokinase activity to fall slightly, whereas galactose feeding supplemented the activity. In the gut and kidney the activity of galactokinase shows a fall in activity in postnatal life that is similar to the liver pattern. Since the effect of galactose or its deprivation was tested only during the declining phase of the postnatal enzyme pattern, it is difficult to interpret the significance of these results in terms of the initial inductive mechanisms for hepatic galactokinase, but, since the enzyme is already present in the late fetal liver, it is certainly not possible to implicate galactose in its initial induction from the available evidence.

### Alanine Aminotransferase (EC 2.6.1.2) and Aspartate Aminotransferases (EC 2.6.1.1)

The prenatal and postnatal pattern of activity for both enzymes has been determined for rat liver (Kafer and Pollack, 29; Nakata, Suematsu, and Sakamoto, 39; Yeung and Oliver, 59). Although there are some differences in the data from these several authors, there is no doubt that—

   (a) the specific activities of the mitochondrial forms of the enzymes do not change significantly from the late fetal liver through the first 20 postnatal days;
   (b) there is a sixfold rise in the cytoplasmic aspartate transaminase activity over the first 10 days after birth and a slow decline thereafter;
   (c) the cytoplasmic activity of alanine aminotransferase shows little change over the first 18 postnatal days and thereafter rises slowly.

It is apparent from all the data that both the mitochondrial and the cytoplasmic forms of the enzymes are already present in the late fetal liver. In a study on weanling rats of unstated age (presumably older than 20 days) Radhakrishnamurty and Sabry (44) studied the effect of pyridoxine deprivation on the levels of both enzymes in liver and erythrocytes. The pyridoxine deficient diets were given for 64 days and the enzyme activities compared with controls pair-fed over the same period. Most of the activities reported were measured in the absence of added pyridoxal phosphate and therefore reflect only holoenzyme activity. It is thus not surprising to find that pyridoxine deficiency resulted in a decline of cytoplasmic transaminase activity over the 64-day period of deprivation. Liver mitochrondrial (holoenzyme) activity, however, did not decline. Assays of activity in the presence of pyridoxal phosphate, which were done in one experiment with aspartate aminotransferase, showed that a 60-day period of pyridoxine deficiency did not significantly alter the content of total enzyme in either liver cytoplasm or mitochondria, but there was a significant depression ($P \leq 0.01$) of total enzyme content in erythrocytes. This study illustrates an important point of methodology. Levels of both holoenzyme and total enzyme must be measured in studies involving cofactor deprivation in order to distinguish effects of cofactor availability to the enzyme from effects on the steady-state levels of enzyme protein. In addition, studies such as those described yield no information on the role of cofactor in the initial induction of enzyme sythesis.

### UDP-Glucuronyl Transferase (EC 2.4.1.17)

The glucuronide-forming system in the liver and kidney of fetal and newborn animals of some species is much less active than in the adult tissues (for bibliography see Kretchmer et al., 34). In some strains of the Dutch rabbit the activity in the liver is 0 to 20% of the adult value, and Flint, Lathe, and Ricketts (14) used this species to examine the effect of food deprivation on enzyme development. Newborn animals were parted from their mothers for a period of 16 hours each day and this treatment was continued for four to nine days. Such treatment consistently retarded the normal postnatal increase in glucuronyl transferase activity, whereas dietary supplementation with an amino acid concentrate had no effect on the extent of normal enzyme development. The effect of partial starvation is consistent with the occurrence of *de novo* enzyme synthesis in the neonatal period but the results of the experiment are not definitive as far as initiation of synthesis are concerned. It is, of course, hardly surprising that partial starvation should result in a slower rate of enzyme development, but the authors also tested the effects of a wide range of hormones and some other substances in an attempt to identify potential inducers or inhibitors of enzyme synthesis. All these agents were without effect on postnatal enzyme development. In this system there again appears to be no clue to the nature of the enzyme-inductive events.

### Pyruvate Kinase (EC 2.7.1.40)

The total activity of pyruvate kinase in neonatal rat liver has been shown to remain at a constant level for about 20 postnatal days and then to increase threefold to sixfold over a relatively short period of a few days (Taylor, Bailey, and Bartley, 53; Vernon and Walker, 54, 55). This increase in activity corresponds to the time at which the carbohydrate content in the neonatal rat diet increases because of weaning. Accordingly, the two groups of authors have tested the effects of weaning to diets differing in the content of fat, carbohydrate, and protein. The results obtained by each group were similar in that the increase in pyruvate kinase activity that occurred on weaning to stock diets did not occur when high fat diets were used. In the experiments of Vernon and Walker (55) it was also shown that premature weaning to high fat or high protein diets prevented the increase that results from preweaning to a high glucose diet. This system, however, also shows somewhat similar characteristics to the glucokinase system previously discussed; for example, young rats weaned to a high glucose diet at 18 or 21 days show a sixfold rise in hepatic pyruvate kinase activity over the next three days, whereas the administration of high glucose milk from day 12 to day 15 yields no increase. In other words, the enzyme system responds to high glucose administration at day 18 or 21 but does not respond at earlier ages. It appears unlikely that changes in alimentation can account for these findings, since the dietary carbohydrate was glucose and not a complex polysaccharide, but some related evidence suggests that this effect may be an insulin-mediated induction of enzyme in response to dietary glucose with characteristics similar to the glucokinase system; that is, that the neonatal liver is unable to respond in this specific way to insulin until about the sixteenth to eighteenth postnatal day.

Tanaka, Harano, Morimura, and Mori (52) reported the presence of at least two distinct forms of pyruvate kinase in adult rat liver. The enzyme forms could be resolved by starch block electrophoresis. One form had the electrophoretic mobility of muscle pyruvate kinase (M), which appears to be a single enzyme, and the other form was called the L-form. Although in the original report intermediate forms also appeared to exist, a later publication (Suda, 50) shows only two well-defined electrophoretic peaks called M and L. The L-form of liver was shown by Tanaka et al. (52) to be under dietary regulation, but from experiments with alloxan diabetic rats and effects of insulin and dietary treatment they came to the conclusion that the dietary effects were mediated via insulin. The L-form but not the M-form of the enzyme appears to require insulin at least for its maintenance in adult rat liver. The two forms have also been shown to be serologically, chemically, and kinetically distinct (Tanaka et al., 52; Suda, 50). Thus it is quite likely that the dramatic increase in pyruvate kinase activity shown in the neonatal rat liver in response to glucose administration and weaning is due to the initial induction of pyruvate kinase L and that the previously apparent activity is due to the M-form. If this is so, then the system would be a rewarding one to study from the point of view of both hormonal and dietary mechanisms in initial induction. Suda (50) made brief mention that "the type M enzyme was also predominant in regenerating or fetal liver." Thus the system in the neonatal animals should be further analyzed.

## ATP-Citrate Lyase (EC 4.1.3.6)

This enzyme is concerned in processes of lipogenesis and, although hepatic activity is readily detectable in fetal and newborn rats, the activity falls off to low levels between postnatal days 10 and 20 and thereafter shows a rapid rise (Taylor et al., 53; Ballard and Hanson, 1; Vernon and Walker, 54, 55). Studies on the effects of weaning show that a high fat diet retards the subsequent development of activity (Taylor et al., 1967; Vernon and Walker, 55) while weaning to a high protein diet has the same effect (Vernon and Walker, 55). Weaning to a high glucose diet potentiates somewhat the normal rise in activity shown in stock diet weanlings (Vernon and Walker, 55). The postnatal changes in enzyme activity show a pattern that is consistent with the weaning-period induction of a new form of the enzyme and perhaps this system should also be analysed for such a phenomenon as suggested for the pyruvate kinase system.

## NADP-Malate Dehydrogenase ("Malic" Enzyme) (EC 1.1.1.40)

This enzyme catalyses the decarboxylation and oxidation of malate to pyruvate and $CO_2$ and is found in liver cytoplasm. It is thus different from the mitochrondrial NAD-malic dehydrogenase. The enzyme is probably absent from the fetal and neonatal rat liver and certainly its activity is extremely low even during the second and third weeks of postnatal life. Activity rises sharply after the twentieth postnatal day (Ballard and Hanson, 1; Taylor et al., 53; Vernon and Walker, 54, 55). Some evidence is presented that preweaning at days 16 and 17 to high glucose diets results in some degree of precocious development of the enzyme, but the results of weaning experiments to high protein and high fat (Vernon and Walker, 55) appear to be inconsistent. In a further paper on this enzyme in brown adipose tissue (Hemon and Berbey, 22) somewhat similar effects of different diets in weanling rats were reported. A high fat diet is effective in maintaining the level of enzyme activity at the preweaning level, but a high carbohydrate diet causes increases to occur. On weaning to high carbohydrate diets increases in the liver enzyme were more sensitive to thyroxin treatment, which potentiated the response to carbohydrate intake. Although this enzyme system may well be a desirable one for study of inductive effects of dietary change the reported results do not yield any particularly lucid clues to the role of such changes in the enzyme induction.

### Tyrosine Aminotransferase (EC 2.6.1.5)

The postnatal induction of tyrosine aminotransferase in rat liver, already mentioned, is not brought about by access of the newborn animal to food, since surgically delivered rats maintained alone in a humidicrib still produce the enzyme (Holt and Oliver, 23, 24), and the time course of enzyme accumulation in the liver is not significantly different in premature starved animals and naturally born fed animals (Holt and Oliver, 23). It has in fact been claimed that denial of food may be a physiological condition for newborn animals that is essential for induction of the enzyme. Premature and full-term rats all go through a phase of intense but transient hypoglycaemia (see Yeung and Oliver, 61, for quantitative details of the rat), and Greengard and Dewey (19) suggested that such hypoglycaemia is a physiological trigger for the enzyme induction. They reported that glucose injections given at birth to vaginally delivered animals resulted in repression of postnatal synthesis of the transaminase. Holt and Oliver (23), however, were unable to confirm this finding in surgically delivered littermate animals to which injections of glucose and some other hexoses were made within 10 minutes of delivery. Instead they showed that repression was apparent only when glucose injections were given two and a half hours after delivery, at the time when the blood glucose is at its lowest level. Since the natural delivery of a rat litter may take as long as two hours, these results are not inconsistent with those of Greengard and Dewey (19) if the latter authors began glucose injections only after the delivery of all the animals in each litter. Such experimental details are not clarified in their paper.

Greengard and Dewey (19) and subsequently Greengard (18) have suggested that postnatal hypoglycaemia promotes release of pancreatic glucagon which is then the hormonal inducer of postnatal synthesis of tyrosine aminotransferase. Holt and Oliver (23, 24) have pointed up anomalies to this hypothesis and have recently shown that the enzyme occurs in multiple forms. Different hormones specifically stimulate or induce the production of the different forms (Holt and Oliver, 25). There is, in addition, good evidence to implicate adrenal cortical hormones in postnatal induction of the enzyme (Sereni et al., 48; Holt and Oliver, 24) and the system is undoubtedly complex. In this case there is little doubt that hormonal factors are of prime importance in postnatal initial induction of the enzyme and that dietary factors (e.g., early exposure to glucose or other hexoses) in fact retard the process of enzyme induction. Although the details of the postnatal hormonal induction mechanisms are still not clear, it is most likely that glucose administration inhibits glucagon release which is involved in some complex way with the inductive mechanisms.

## Phosphopyruvate Carboxylase (EC 4.1.1.32)

The fetal rat liver is incapable of the synthesis of glucose or glycogen from pyruvate or amino acids (gluconeogenesis), but the overall metabolic pathway develops within a few hours of natural or surgical delivery (Ballard and Oliver, 3; Yeung and Oliver, 59, 60). The overall capacity for gluconeogenesis is due to the rapid postnatal synthesis of a single enzyme which is an obligatory catalytic component of the metabolic pathway. This cytoplasmic enzyme, phosphopyruvate carboxylase, is absent from the fetal liver (Yeung and Oliver, 60; Ballard and Hanson, 2) and makes its appearance only after birth. Experiments with inhibitors of DNA-directed RNA-synthesis and protein synthesis indicate that the enzyme is synthesized *de novo* and the system is a good example of initial induction. In this system Yeung and Oliver (61, 62) have shown that postnatal hypoglycaemia is the essential physiological trigger to the induction mechanism, but in addition there is a backup system involving catecholamines. The suggested mechanism (Yeung and Oliver, 62) is that hypoglycaemia promotes the release of pancreatic glucagon which then stimulates the production of 3′,5′-cyclic adenosine monophosphate in the liver (Sutherland and Robinson, 51). Cyclic AMP appears to be the intracellular effector molecule for the induction of the enzyme. Cyclic AMP, glucagon, adrenalin, and noradrenalin are all effective inducers for the enzyme when administered to the rat fetus *in utero*. In the normal postnatal induction of the enzyme glucose injections in amounts sufficient to prevent hypoglycaemia result in as much as 80% repression of enzyme synthesis but are never totally effective in preventing all synthesis. Adrenergic blockage agents also repress postnatal enzyme synthesis but are similarly only partly effective. Thus postnatal production of catecholamines also appears to be part of the physiological induction mechanism and these compounds, too, stimulate cyclic

AMP production in the liver (Sutherland and Robinson, 51). The catecholamine mechanism is apparently the backup system which results in enzyme induction even when hypoglycaemia is completely prevented.

The rate of enzyme production in surgically delivered starved animals is the same as in naturally delivered animals which remain with the mother (Yeung and Oliver, 60). This is probably because female rats do not feed their young for some time after delivery of the whole litter is complete. The prompt administration of glucose at birth has quite dramatic inhibitory effects on enzyme synthesis, but it is clear that the results of such "nutritional" manipulation are not due to some direct action of glucose as a repressor of enzyme synthesis. The effects are best explained as being due to the prevention of hypoglycaemia and the consequent reduction in glucagon output. Thus the change in the dietary environment at birth is mediated by humoral agents whose effects in turn are mediated at the intracellular level by a small molecular effector—in this case cyclic AMP.

## METHODOLOGICAL PROBLEMS

The dietary manipulation of postnatal animals is difficult and tedious to arrange, especially with the laboratory rat. Stomach intubation or eyedropper hand feeding is time consuming, especially when large numbers of animals are needed. A recent technique for artificial feeding of infant rats by continuous gastric infusion (Messer, Thoman, Terrasa, and Dallman, 37) promises to remove the tedium from hand rearing and to allow the administration of any chosen dietary regime under strictly controlled conditions. In this technique infant rats are maintained in a humidicrib and connected via an indwelling gastric cannula and tubing to a slow injection pump. The authors have inserted the gastric cannula as early as four hours after birth and maintained animals at normal growth rates for 20 days. One of the authors is said to have worked on the project in order to enjoy the delights of San Francisco evenings rather than spending his time wet nursing the entire infant rat colony (Dr. M. Messer, private communication).

In neonatal animals the interpretation of nutritional effects may be complicated by changes in alimentation. The absorptive capacity of the gut is known to change (e.g., Jordan and Morgan, 28; Batt and Schachter, 5), as is its spectrum of digestive enzymes during neonatal development (e.g., Doell and Kretchmer, 10, 11).

In this review we have attempted to assess the evidence of nutritional effects on enzyme development which we defined as the initial induction of enzyme protein synthesis. The systems in which such events take place must be identified, and some problems are encountered. The use of antisera to the induced enzyme may allow detection of enzyme protein even before activity appears in the tissue, and because of its specificity this procedure is probably the method of choice to allow identification of the time at which induction of specific protein synthesis begins. Many enzymes, however, are not available in a state of antigenic purity and so antisera cannot be prepared. In these cases inhibitors of RNA synthesis and of protein synthesis ars used to identify the nature of the apparent induction. All the commonly used agents, but especially actinomycin D, puromycin, and cycloheximide, are cytotoxic, and apparent inhibition of enzyme production may be due to morbidity in the experimental animal. In our laboratory neonatal rats appear to tolerate actinomycin D at doses to 1 $\mu$g/g body weight and puromycin to 150 $\mu$g/g body weight for periods up to eight hours, but some surgically delivered animals become inactive over the first few hours with actinomycin D and doses need to be decreased to about 0.5 $\mu$g/g to maintain activity. The higher dose is just sufficient to block the postnatal synthesis of phosphopyruvate carboxylase and tyrosine aminotransferase, but at the lower dose inhibition of synthesis is incomplete. After the identification of the time of initial induction dietary manipulation before and during the event should reveal the operation of nutritional factors. If such factors are involved in physiological induction, they should be capable of the precocious evocation of the induced event. Some presently known systems that should be stimulating and rewarding to study include the postnatal induction of glucokinase and NADP-malate dehydrogenase. Should analysis of the ATP-citrate lyase and pyruvate kinase systems reveal the induction of specific isozymes when the large increase in activity occurs at the twentieth postnatal day, these systems, too, would be rewarding of study. These developmental events have been suggested because nutritional changes can be readily made well before the inductive event takes place.

## CONCLUSIONS

The experimental work that has been reviewed offers no clear evidence of the operation of nutrients as primary factors in enzyme development, nor is there evidence that dietary manipulation can prevent or modify significantly the qualitative aspects of enzyme development, although quantitative responses may be affected. Nutrients, however, may represent stimuli that trigger the release of humoral agents which are themselves the intracellular effectors for enzyme induction or which in their turn promote the production of, or are converted to, the specific intracellular effectors.

## APOLOGIA

The authors seek absolution in advance for their sins of omission, both grave and trivial, and for their restricted definition of enzyme development. This restricted view was adopted largely because we are developmentalists rather than nutritionalists and by this device we enjoyed the luxury of a brief article.

## REFERENCES

1. F. J. Ballard and R. W. Hanson, *Biochem. J.* **102**: 952 (1967).
2. F. J. Ballard and R. W. Hanson, *Biochem. J.* **104**: 866 (1967).
3. F. J. Ballard and I. T. Oliver, *Biochim. Biophys. Acta* **71**: 578 (1963).
4. F. J. Ballard and I. T. Oliver, *Bochem. J.* **90**: 261 (1964).
5. E. R. Batt and D. Schachter, *Amer. J. Physiol.* **216**: 1064 (1969).
6. P. Cuatrecasas and S. Segal, *J. Biol. Chem.* **240**: 2382 (1965).
7. V. E. Davis, *Endocrinology* **72**: 33 (1963).
8. D. L. Dipietro, C. Sharma, and S. Weinhouse, *Biochemistry,* **1**: 455 (1962).
9. D. L. Dipietro and S. Weinhouse, *J. Biol. Chem.* **235**: 2542 (1960).
10. R. Doell and N. Kretchmer, *Biochim. Biophys. Acta* **67**: 516 (1963).
11. R. Doell and N. Kretchmer, *Science* **143**: 42 (1964).
12. E. D. Eberle and S. Eiduson, *J. Neurochem.* **15**: 1071 (1968).
13. P. Feigelson, T. Dashman, and F. Margolis, *Arch. Biochem. Biophys.* **85**: 478 (1958).
14. M. Flint, G. H. Lathe, and J. R. Ricketts, *Ann. N.Y. Acad. Sci.* **111**: 295 (1963).
15. L. Goldstein, E. J. Stella, and W. E. Knox, *J. Biol. Chem.* **237**: 1723 (1962).
16. A. I. Grayzel, P. Horchner, and I. London, *Proc. Natl. Acad. Sci. (USA),* **55**: 650 (1966).
17. O. Greengard, in *Advances in Enzyme Regulation,* G. Weber, Ed. New York: Pergamon, Vol. 1, 1963, p. 61.
18. O. Greengard, *Science* **163**: 891 (1969).
19. O. Greengard and H. K. Dewey, *J. Biol. Chem.* **242**: 2986 (1967).
20. O. Greengard and P. Feigelson, *J. Biol. Chem.* **236**: 158 (1961).
21. O. Greengard, and P. Feigelson, *Nature* **190**: 446 (1961).

22. P. Hemon, and B. Berbey, *Biochim. Biophys. Acta* **170**: 235 (1968).

23. P. G. Holt and I. T. Oliver, *Biochem. J.* **108**: 333 (1968).

24. P. G. Holt and I. T. Oliver, *Biochemistry* **8**: 1429 (1969).

25. P. G. Holt and I. T. Oliver, *FEBS Letters* **5**: 89 (1969).

25a. P. G. Holt and I. T. Oliver, *Inter. J. Biochem.* **2**: 212 (1971).

26. D. Holten, W. D. Wicks, and F. T. Kenney, *J. Biol. Chem.* **242**: 1053 (1967).

27. F. Jacob and J. Monod, *J. Mol. Biol.* **3**: 318 (1961).

28. S. M. Jordan and E. H. Morgan, *Aust. J. Exptl. Biol. Med. Sci.* **46**: 465 (1968).

29. E. Kafer and J. K. Pollack, *Exp. Cell Res.* **22**: 120 (1961).

30. F. T. Kenney and W. L. Albritton, *Proc. Natl. Acad. Sci. (USA)* **54**: 1693 (1966).

31. F. T. Kenney and R. M. Flora, *J. Biol. Chem.* **236**: 2699 (1961).

32. W. E. Knox, in *Advances in Enzyme Regulation* G. Weber, Ed. New York: Pergamon, Vol. 4, 1966, p. 287.

33. W. E. Knox and V. H. Auerbach, *J. Biol. Chem.* **214**: 307 (1955).

34. N. Kretcher, R. E. Greenberg, and F. Sereni, *Ann. Rev. Med.* **14**: 407 (1963).

35. E. C. C. Lin and W. E. Knox, *Biochim. Biophys. Acta* **26**: 85 (1957).

36. G. Litwack and A. M. Nemeth, *Arch. Biochem. Biophys.* **109**: 316 (1965).

37. M. Messer, E. B. Thoman, A. G. Terrasa, and P. R. Dallman, *J. Nutr.* **98**: 404 (1969).

38. S. A. Miller, in *Mammalian Protein Metabolism,* H. N. Munro, Ed. New York: Academic, Vol. III, 1969, p. 183.

39. Y. Nakata, T. Suematsu, and Y. Sakamoto, *J. Biochem. (Tokyo)*, **55**: 199 (1964).

40. A. M. Nemeth, *J. Biol. Chem.* **234**: 2021 (1959).

41. A. M. Nemeth, *Ann. N.Y. Acad. Sci.* **111**: 199 (1963).

42. H. Niemeyer, L. Clark-Turri, and E. Rabille, *Nature* **198**: 1096 (1963).

43. H. C. Pitot and Y. S. Cho, *Cold Spring Harbour Symp. Quant. Biol.* **26**: 371 (1961).

44. R. Radhakrishnamurty and Z. I. Sabry, *Canad. J. Biochem.* **46**: 1081 (1968).

45. F. Rosen and H. Milholland, *J. Biol. Chem.* **238**: 3730 (1963).

46. M. Salas, E. Vinuella, and A. Sols, *J. Biol. Chem.* **238**: 3535 (1963).

47. R. T. Schimke, *Bull. Soc. Chim. Biol.* **48**: 1009 (1966).

48. F. Sereni, F. T. Kenney, and N. Kretchmer, *J. Biol. Chem.* **234**: 609 (1959).

49. C. Sharma, R. Manjeshwar, and S. Weinhouse, *J. Biol. Chem.* **238**: 3840 (1963).

50. M. Suda, in *Advances in Enzyme Regulation,* G. Weber, Ed. New York: Pergamon, Vol. 5, 1967, p. 181.

51. E. W. Sutherland and G. A. Robinson, *Pharmacol. Rev.* **18**: 145 (1966).

52. T. Tanaka, Y. Harano, H. Morimura, and R. Mori, *Biochem. Biophys. Res. Comm.* **21**: 55 (1965).

53. C. B. Taylor, E. Bailey, and W. Bartley, *Biochem. J.* **105**: 717 (1967).

54. R. G. Vernon and D. G. Walker, *Biochem. J.* **106**: 321 (1968).

55. R. C. Vernon and D. G. Walker, *Biochem. J.* **106**: 331 (1968).

56. D. G. Walker, *Biochim. Biophys. Acta* **77**: 209 (1963).

57. D. G. Walker and G. Holland, *Biochem. J.* **97**: 845 (1965).

58. O. Wiss and F. Weber, *Vitamins and Hormones* **22**: 495 (1964).

59. D. Yeung and I. T. Oliver, *Biochem. J.* **103**: 744 (1967).

60. D. Yeung and I. T. Oliver, *Biochem. J.* **105**: 1229 (1967).

61. D. Yeung and I. T. Oliver, *Biochem. J.* **108**: 325 (1968).

62. D. Yeung and I. T. Oliver, *Biochemistry* **7**: 3231 (1968).

# 3

## Nutrition and Cell Growth

MYRON WINICK, M.D.

Professor of Pediatrics and Director of the Institute of Human Nutrition

JO ANNE BRASEL, M.D.

Associate Professor of Pediatrics

PEDRO ROSSO, M.D.

Adjunct Assistant Professor of Public Health Nutrition, Columbia University College of Physicians and Surgeons

Growth of any organ may be caused by an increase in the number of cells, by an increase in the size of already existing cells, or by both increases occurring simultaneously. The total number of cells can be measured by determining the total organ DNA content and dividing by a constant which represents the DNA content per diploid nucleus in the species being studied (13, 38); for example, all diploid rat cells contain 6.2 pg of DNA and all diploid human cells contain 6.0 pg of DNA. Except for a few tetraploid Purkinje cells in the cerebellum and in the cerebral cortex, all the cells making up the mammalian brain are diploid (66). Thus, for practical purposes, total brain DNA content represents the total number of brain cells, and total cerebellar or cerebral DNA represents the total number of cells in each of those regions. In the liver the existence of ploidy makes these measurements more difficult to interpret. Epstein has shown, however, that as ploidy increases the cytoplasmic mass of the cell increases proportionally (40). Thus a tetraploid liver cell nucleus governs twice as much cytoplasm as a diploid

49

liver nucleus. Liver growth therefore can be examined by using the same principles as long as it is kept in mind that although a doubling of the chromosome number will double the nuclear DNA content it may not result in two discrete nuclei. The cytoplasm will also double in size but will not divide into separate cells.

Certain other organs, such as skeletal muscle and aging pancreas, contain a significant proportion of multinuclear cells (39). In these organs an increase in DNA content represents an increase in nuclear number and not an increase in the actual number of cells. If we assume that each nucleus governs a discrete, though not bounded, cytoplasmic mass, then the same principles may be employed. Finally, certain organs contain diploid nuclei but no discrete cell boundaries. These organs are true syncytia. Placenta in most species is such an organ. Again, the same principles are operable if we assume that each nucleus governs a discrete cytoplasmic mass.

Once the number of cells is determined, the average weight per cell, protein content per cell, RNA content per cell, or lipid content per cell can be determined simply by analyzing for the total amount of each of these components and dividing by the number of cells. The result can be expressed chemically as a weight/DNA, protein/DNA, RNA/DNA, or lipid/DNA ratio. Thus, regardless of whether actual cell number or "cell mass" is calculated, the thesis that increase in total organ DNA content represents one aspect of growth, namely, an increase in the number of cells, whereas an increase in the weight/DNA or protein/DNA ratio and, in certain cases, the lipid/DNA ratio represents another aspect of growth, namely, increase in mass without increase in cell number, would appear to be valid.

Note that total DNA content, although accurately reflecting cell number, in no way differentiates one cell type from another. In addition, although the ratios as outlined above give an overall average for these materials per cell, no single cell may actually contain this quantity of material. Individual cells, especially when differing in type, may vary widely in their composition of protein, RNA, or lipids. Within these limitations, however, this "chemical" approach to growth has allowed us to make certain generalizations which have given rise to an overall picture of growth on a cellular level.

## GENERAL CONSIDERATIONS

Early growth in the rat proceeds entirely by cell division. DNA, weight, and protein all increase proportionally to a constant cell size which is expressed by a weight/DNA or a protein/DNA ratio (111). The rate of DNA synthesis, and therefore of cell division, decreases at different times for different organs. Protein content continues its initial rise, which results in an increased protein/DNA ratio. Increase in cell size, then, occurs not as a consequence of increased rates of protein accumulation but as a consequence of decreased rates of cell division. If the weight/DNA ratio is used to assess cell size, the same relationships hold as for protein, except during the neonatal period, when weight/DNA ratios either remain constant or decrease. This suggests that a loss of water occurs during the neonatal period, an observation that has been made in many animals, including the human (58).

Slowing of growth with approaching maturity is due to the attainment of a steady state between protein synthesis and destruction. Note that DNA synthesis stops in most organs before the organ has attained its maximum weight or protein content (111). For the rat and most of its organs growth from 10 days after conception to maturity can be divided into three phases. The first consists of rapid cell division in which cell size remains constant; the second consists of an increase in cell number and size as both DNA and protein content rise, but as a result of a decrease in the rate of DNA synthesis protein rises out of proportion to DNA; the third consists of an increase in cell size as DNA synthesis stops and protein continues to accumulate. Growth finally ceases when protein synthesis and degradation come into equilibrium. These phases do not change abruptly but merge gradually, one into the other (111).

The organs of the lymphoid system exhibit a very different pattern of growth. In both spleen and thymus weight/DNA and protein/DNA ratios remain constant. Growth in these organs occurs by cell division without increase in cell size. It is interesting that of all the organs studied these two are the renewing type with a rapid cell turnover (111).

Total organ RNA increases during growth. Except in liver, this increase is always proportional to the increase in DNA and results in an RNA/DNA ratio that is constant in the particular organ and does not vary with time. Certain tissues, such as liver, heart, and skeletal muscle, show high RNA/DNA ratios, whereas tissues such as spleen and thymus show low ratios. These relationships are similar to the protein/DNA ratios finally shown by these tissues. These data tend to reinforce the concept that tissues most actively engaged in protein synthesis are rich in RNA. The high RNA/DNA ratio, however, occurs early in development, long before the high protein/DNA ratios are reached in the same tissues. Skeletal muscle, heart, and salivary gland are good examples of this phenomenon. RNA/DNA ratios are high but do not change significantly from 4 to 44 days. Protein/DNA ratios, however, increase markedly during that period. It would appear that during early growth RNA reaches its final amount per cell even in the face of rapid cell division and that this amount is sufficient to sustain normal rates of protein synthesis (111). Liver appears to be one exception. Our data indicate an increase in the RNA/DNA ratio in liver during the neonatal period (111). These results correlate with increased enzymatic activity occurring at that time (78).

These data allow us to view the overall growth of an organ as a continuous accretion of protoplasm made up of water, proteins, RNA, and, in some cases, lipids. The ultimate arrangement of this protoplasm into individual cells depends on the rate of DNA synthesis. At present the mechanisms controlling the period during which DNA may be synthesized by an organ and the mechanisms governing the rate of synthesis during that period are largely unknown. In recent years some insight into these problems has been achieved. The time during the growing period when cells are actively proliferating in any organ is under genetic control. This time will vary tremendously in different species; for example, in the rat brain cell division is over by day 21 postnatally (111). In the guinea pig there is very little cell division in brain after birth. In contrast, in the human brain cell division continues until around the end of the first year of life (103).

How then does the gene "turn off" cell division in the various organs of a particular species? If, as is currently thought, gene action involves the control of protein synthesis, we may assume that the synthesis or lack of synthesis of a particular protein under "genetic direction" will, at least in part, control the rate of cell division. The enzyme DNA polymerase may be essential for the final synthesis of DNA. Recently it has been shown that the activity of this enzyme mimics the rate of DNA synthesis in chick brain (73) and in rat brain (16). In rat brain the maximum rate of DNA synthesis is achieved at about 10 days of age. Enzyme activity, with either native or denatured calf thymus DNA as a primer, peaks at 6 to 10 days of age (Fig. 1). Moreover, activity is highest in those regions in which cell division is most rapid.[*] Whether control of the activity of this enzyme is the primary mechanism by which the gene regulates the rate of cell division or a secondary mechanism is yet to be determined.

Most of the work on normal cellular growth in various organs is still largely descriptive. This descriptive approach, however, has not only allowed for some research into control mechanisms but has also provided

---

[*] J. A. Brasel, B. S. Joh, R. A. Ehrenkranz, and M. Winick, unpublished data.

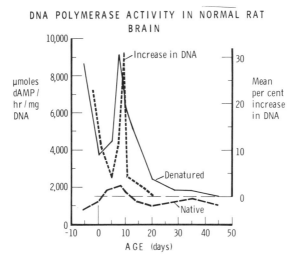

DNA POLYMERASE ACTIVITY IN NORMAL RAT BRAIN

**Fig. 1.** DNA polymerase activity per milligram of DNA in normal rat brain and mean percent increase in DNA per day. Reprinted from J. A. Brasel, R. A. Ehrenkranz, and Myron Winick, "DNA Polymerase Activity in Rat Brain during Ontogeny." *Develop. Biol.* **23**, 424, (1970).

new tools to assess the effects of numerous growth-retarding stimuli on the cellular growth of different organs. In the remainder of this chapter we consider the normal growth of the brain and the effects of altered nutrition on that growth. In addition, we review what is known about normal growth of certain other tissues and how that growth is influenced by the state of nutrition. Finally, we consider prenatal nutritional influences on the cellular growth of both placenta and fetal brain.

## NORMAL CELLULAR GROWTH OF VARIOUS TISSUES

### Brain

Detailed examination of normal cellular growth in rat brain reveals that different regions undergo different patterns of growth. In cerebrum DNA synthesis continues until about 21 days postnatally (72). After that the cells continue to accumulate protein and lipid. Total cerebral lipid content is achieved somewhat later, and total protein content at about 99 days of age. In cerebellum DNA synthesis stops at 17 days postnatally. Net protein synthesis actually becomes negative for a short period after that, and the size of the individual cerebellar cells decreases. This decrease in cell size in cerebellum with age probably reflects the maturation of larger more primitive cells into smaller more mature cells. In brain stem the total cell number increases to 14 days of age. Thereafter there is an enormous increase in the protein/DNA ratio which probably reflects not only an increase in the size of the brain-stem cells but also ingrowth, myelination, and extension of neuronal processes from other brain regions into the brain stem. Hippocampus demonstrates a type of cellular growth unique to the central nervous system. There is a discrete rise in DNA content between the fourteenth and seventeenth days of life (42), an increase that corresponds to a migration of neurons from under the lateral venticle into the hippocampus which occurs on the fifteenth day after birth in the rat (3, 5).

The ultimate cellular makeup of the various regions depends, then, on the rate of cell division within the particular region, the time that cell division stops, the type of cells dividing, and whether the cells are migrating to or from the region.

The sequence of events is not so clearly defined in human brain as in rat brain (32, 59, 103). Studies in our laboratory indicate that DNA synthesis is linear prenatally, begins to slow down shortly after birth, and reaches a maximum at about 8 to 12 months of age (103) (Fig. 2). More recent studies have modified these results somewhat and extend the time beyond the first year of life. Moreover, Dobbing and Sands have shown that two peaks of DNA synthesis may occur normally in the human brain. The first peak is reached at about 26 weeks of gestation and the second around birth (32) (Fig. 3). They have interpreted these

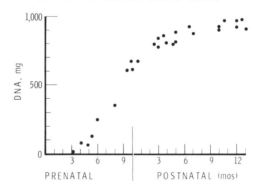

DNA CONTENT OF NORMAL HUMAN BRAIN

**Fig. 2.**   Total DNA content of the human brain derived from 27 cases of therapeutic abortions, crib deaths, accidental deaths, and poisonings. Reprinted from *Fed. Proc.* **29**, 1511 (1970).

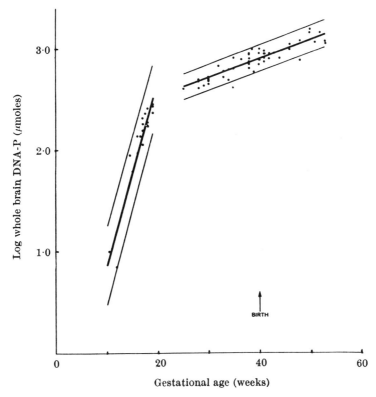

**Fig. 3.** The logarithm of whole brain DNA in developing human brain. Reprinted from *Nature* **226**, 639 (1970).

results as corresponding to the peak rate of neuronal division and the peak rate of glial division, respectively.

Note that Brasel et al. have reported two peaks in DNA polymerase activity in developing rat brain (see Fig. 1), one occurring prenatally and one between 6 and 10 days postnatally (16). It is possible that the rate of neuronal cell division is most rapid prenatally and that the first peak reflects that rate.

There are still very few data on the cellular growth of various regions of the human brain. Available data indicate that the rate of cell division postnatally is about the same in cerebrum and cerebellum and stops at about the same time in both areas, that is, between 12 and 15 months of age (116). The number of cases studied, however, is too small to determine the exact time at which cell division stops in these areas.

In brain stem DNA synthesis continues at a slow but rather steady rate until at least 1 year of age (116). Here, again, cell types involved and the migratory patterns of the cells in the developing human brain are not so clearly worked out as in rat brain. For obvious reasons radio-autography cannot be done. What is known is the result of careful histological and histochemical examination of the brains of fetuses of various ages. In a series of elegant studies (33, 34, 35, 36) Duckett and Pearse have shown that during fetal life the brain not only increases linearly in weight but undergoes a series of biochemical changes. Glycolysis is present during the second month of fetal life; oxidative mechanisms appear during the third month; and activity and localization of a number of enzymes reach a mature pattern during the seventh month of fetal life.

In addition there is evidence that the presence of acetylcholinesterase indicates tissue excitability (75). The activity of this enzyme is localized in neurones of the anterior horn of the spinal cord as early as the tenth week of embryonic life. This correlates well with the time that movement of the lower limbs can be elicited by proper stimulation (8).

Two specific cell types, the Cajal-Retzius cells (35) and the monamine oxidase cells (34), are present only in fetal life, disappearing before birth. Their function is unknown.

Not only is the brain composed of a multiplicity of cell types but it is a unique organ in yet another way. Its cells contain DNA, RNA, and proteins and many of them also contain relatively large amounts of lipid. The major components of brain lipids are simple lipids, such as cholesterol and fatty acids, and compound lipids, such as phospholipids, glycolipids, and other esters. Although most of the lipid is contained within cell membranes (e.g., myelin sheaths), some is contained in other subcellular fractions such as endoplasmic reticulum and mitochondria. Since the bulk of the total brain lipid is present as a component of myelin, changes in lipids during development constitute changes in myelination.

Cholesterol is the only sterol present in appreciable amounts in the adult nervous system. In the young animal, however, demosterol and zymosterol have been reported (57, 65). These appear to be precursors of cholesterol. Although most cholesterol in the nervous system is in the free form, fatty acid esters of cholesterol are also present, especially in the young animal (1). There are some data to suggest that another cholesterol ester, cholesterol sulfate, is present in normal brain (81). Only trace amounts of free fatty acids are present in brain, the bulk of the fatty acids existing as esters of compound lipids (88). Phospholipids, which account for 20 to 25% of the dry weight of mammalian brain, are compounds in which phosphatidic acid is combined with a base (either choline or ethanolamine) and a hydroxyamino acid (serine or inositol). These lipids would include lecithins (phosphatidyl choline), cephalins (phosphatidyl ethanolamine), lipositols (phosphatidyl inositol), phosphatidyl serine, plasmalogens (acetal phosphatide), and sphingo-myelins (phosphatidyl sphingosides).

Sphingomyelin is the major phosphosphingolipid in animal tissues. Although it contains phosphorylcholine, it differs from lecithin in that the fatty acid is bound by an amide linkage to sphingosine. The di-phosphoinositides and triphosphoinositides, although present only in small amounts, are important in assessing myelination, since they are highly concentrated in the myelin sheath.

Glycolipids exist primarily in two forms, cerebrosides or cerebroside sulfates (sulfatides) and gangliosides. Cerebrosides contain galactose, a high-molecular weight fatty acid, and sphingol or sphingosine (the same complex amino alcohol that is present in sphingomyelin. In the adult brain 90% of the total cerebroside is located within the myelin sheath. Gangliosides are present in lower concentration than cerebro-sides. They consist of N-acetyl neuraminic acid, sphingosine, and three molecules of either glucose or galactose. Gangliosides are found mainly in those areas that contain neurones and are concentrated at nerve end-ings (98).

Total lipid content and concentration increase in whole brain during development. The major increase in concentration occurs in white matter, undoubtedly because progressive myelination is occurring in this area. The rate of total lipid deposition can be used as a measure of the rate of myelin synthesis because of the very slow turnover in the components of myelin in all mammalian species studied so far (67). Most investi-gators have found a marked increase in total lipid content and concentra-tion during the early development of the brain in several mammalian species, including the human (87).

The developmental changes in the major lipid components of rat brain are summarized in Table 1. The rate of cholesterol deposition is maximal between the fifteenth and twentieth days of postnatal growth. This is about one week after the maximal rate of DNA synthesis (30).

In the human there is little change in total lipid composition in either gray or white matter during the first seven months of gestation. There-after lipid deposition proceeds rapidly in gray matter and adult composi-tion is reached at about 3 months of age. In white matter, in which most of the actual myelination is occurring, there is a less rapid lipid deposition. By 2 years of age 90% of the total lipid is deposited and by 10 years of age adult values are attained (14, 28, 89).

Cholesterol concentration increases in both cerebral gray and white

Table 1    Changes in Lipid Composition of the Developing Rat Brain[a]

| | Age (days) | Wet Weight (g) | Choles- terol (mmoles) | Phospho- lipid (mmoles) | Cerebro- sides (mmoles) | Molar Ratio Cholesterol: Phospholipid: Cerebrosides |
|---|---|---|---|---|---|---|
| Whole brain | 10 | 1.00 | 16.00 | 33.60 | 0.18 | 100:210:1 |
| | 16 | 1.25 | 26.90 | 53.00 | 1.25 | 100:197:4.5 |
| | Adult | 1.99 | 96.00 | 119.00 | 22.20 | 100:125:23 |
| Myelin | 10 | 1.00 | 1.47 | 2.07 | 0.077 | 100:140:5 |
| | 16 | — | 3.20 | 4.47 | 0.320 | 100:140:10 |
| | Adult | — | 34.0 | 32.0 | 11.8 | 100:95:35 |

[a] Reprinted from *Applied Neurochemistry*. A. N. Davison and J. Dobbing, Eds. Blackwell Scientific Publications, Oxford and Edinburgh, 1968, p. 273. After Cuzner and Davidson [28].

matter and in cerebellum from early in fetal life (60). In whole brains of fetuses below 2 months of age cholesterol concentration is about 2.38%. The concentration rises to 5.4% at term, 6.65% at 9 months of age, and 10.7% in the adult brain (14). Data on cerebrosides are not clear but suggest an increased concentration in white matter during development (89). All phospholipid fractions increase during development. Phosphatides show little increase after seven months gestation (14, 89). In contrast, cephalin concentration in both white and gray matter increases from 7% at four months gestation to 12% in gray matter and 17% in white matter, the adult levels, by 3 months of age.

Myelination is always preceded by multiplication of oligodendroglial cells (4), following which the glial cells surround the nerve axon in a spiral fashion. After this "wrapping" process is completed there is a progressive deposition of lipids within the sheath (18). Lipids represent about 75% of the dry weight of human myelin. The largest lipid component is cholesterol, but significant amounts of ethanolamine phosphatide, galactolipids, cerebrosides, and cerebroside sulfates are present. The characteristic composition of myelin lipids shows a molar ratio of cholesterol:phospholipid:cerebroside of 2:2:1.

Developmental studies of myelin composition demonstrate considerable changes as lipid deposition progresses. Lecithin decreases in proportion to other phospholipids, whereas cholesterol, phosphatidyl inositol, and ethanolamine phosphatide increase.

Myelin cannot be considered a discrete metabolic entity. The results of [14]C labeling experiments demonstrate that acetic inositol phosphatide, lecithin, and serine phosphatide have much more rapid turnover rates than most of the other components, which show very slow turnover (30). In spite of its relative nonspecificity, cholesterol content has been used in assessing myelination because of its very slow turnover rate and because it is easy to measure.

Serial analysis of lipids in human brains indicates that the lipid/DNA ratio rises from shortly after birth until at least 2 years of age. This is reflected in a rise in the cholesterol/DNA and phospholipid/DNA ratios. Postnatal lipid synthesis is proceeding at a more rapid rate than DNA synthesis, undoubtedly as a result of the rapid myelination that is occurring during this period of life (80).

Recent studies in developing rat brain have shown that during the period of most rapid lipid synthesis glucose is metabolized in much greater proportions through the hexose monophosphate shunt than it is later. More than 50% of glucose metabolism uses this pathway until about 30 days of age; thereafter less than 20% of the metabolism of glucose passes through the shunt. The hexose monophosphate shunt favors both nucleic acid and lipid synthesis. For the former it supplies ribose molecules and for the latter it generates TPNH (106). Human brain has not been studied in this respect. It would be interesting to know whether more glucose is metabolized via the hexose monphosphate shunt pathway in infant brain than in adult brain.

Although the descriptive work in human brain suggests that cellular growth is governed by the same principles as those governing cellular growth in rat brain, more data are needed to complete the picture. Studies investigating the control of cell division in human brain are almost nonexistent. In this respect it should be mentioned that DNA polymerase activity has been measured in human fetal tissue, and it should therefore be possible to determine a developmental curve for this enzyme in human brain.[*]

## Muscle

There have been a number of studies of cellular growth in skeletal muscle of rats (20, 21, 22, 24, 37, 38, 39, 48, 51). Enesco and Puddy (39) determined that 35% of the nuclei in samples of four different limb muscles lay outside the muscle fibers in male Sherman rats at 16, 36, and 86 days of age. Since the percentage of nuclei outside the

[*] J. A. Brasel and E. Velasco, unpublished data.

fiber did not change over the age span studied, an increase in DNA content, even if uncorrected for nonfiber nuclei, will proportionately reflect growth in muscle cell nuclei. This study, in which combined histometric and chemical techniques were used, shows clearly that the number of individual muscle fibers does not increase postnatally but that, despite earlier held concepts, the number of nuclei within the fiber as well as fiber size show significant increments. Note, however, that this study was carried out in normal animals and that the constant percentage of fiber to nonfiber nuclei may not hold true in abnormally growing animals. The DNA content of various striated muscles rises to fixed levels by 90 to 95 days of age, whereas increase in weight, myofibrillar proteins, and sacroplasmic proteins continues until 140 days of age (48). Thus it appears that in the rat hyperplasia of muscle fiber nuclei continues until some 90 days postnatally and hypertrophy of muscle fibers continues to approximately 140 days.

Cheek et al. (22, 25, 51) have also measured total muscle mass and total muscle nuclear number in the Sprague-Dawley rat. Using an ingenious technique, they measured DNA concentration in a sample of skeletal muscle and assessed the total muscle mass from determinations of total noncollagen protein or potassium in pulverized, defatted, dried carcass or from determination of total muscle intracellular water or calcium content of bone. Total muscle nuclear number then equals [(DNA concentration in milligrams per gram) times (muscle mass in grams)] divided by (DNA content per nucleus). The validity of these methods depends on the muscle samples being representative of muscle throughout the body and on the accuracy of noncollagen protein or potassium or intracellular water as reflections of total muscle mass or of calcium content as a reflection of bone mass. These investigators point out that the four different methods give similar results for grams of muscle in normal rats at different ages and that these values are, in turn, similar to values that use creatinine excretion (50) to determine muscle mass and to values obtained by dissection techniques (50). The literature on the constancy of DNA from one muscle to another is contradictory. Although Cheek et al. (24) report agreement for DNA concentration in several muscles of normal male Sprague-Dawley rats and in five muscles studied in young Macaca Mulatta monkeys, Enesco and Puddy (39) find agreement in only certain muscles in male Sherman rats. In addition, there are differences noted with age. In hypophysectomized rats (9), DNA content of various muscles may differ. These data suggest that DNA concentration may vary between different muscle groups, even in the normally growing animal, and therefore that calculation of total muscle nuclear population from the DNA content of a single sample may not provide entirely accurate values, although trends with growth, disease, or therapy might well be assessed in this way. To our knowledge, however, no studies of the constancy of DNA in various muscle groups with malnutrition or overnutrition have been reported. It would seem advisable to perform such studies in whatever abnormal situation is being investigated before relying on these techniques for determination of muscle nuclear number. In the animal these possible pitfalls in methodology can be avoided by removing in toto one or more specific muscles or muscle groups and by measuring directly the weight, DNA, and protein content when studying either normal or abnormal growth. The additional measurement of total muscle mass may possibly give further important information regarding the effects of disease or therapy on muscle growth.

Using the noncollagen protein method, Cheek et al. (50) have measured total muscle mass in normal male and female Sprague-Dawley rats from 3 to 14 weeks of age. In the male muscle mass increases linearly during this period from approximately 15 to 144 g. The female begins with the same amount of 15 g at 3 weeks, but the rate of growth is less rapid, especially after 8 weeks of age. The adult female at 14 weeks achieves a muscle mass of 90 g. These sex differences are erased if muscle mass is compared with total body weight rather than age (50); for example, at a body weight of 200 g both sexes have a muscle mass of approximately 70 g. This study does not document the time of cessation of growth in total muscle mass.

Using indirect methods, Cheek et al. (22, 24) have also assessed growth in muscle "cell mass" during normal growth. Maximum muscle cell mass is reached in normal male Sprague-Dawley rats by 14 weeks, which is slightly earlier than the age noted for the quadriceps muscle by Gordon et al. (48), using total muscle analysis. Normal female rats (22) show similar values to males at 3 weeks; thereafter, until 13 weeks, individual "cell mass" is greater in the female; after 13 weeks the male values exceed the female. This catchup by the male occurs between 8 and 13 weeks (i.e., after cessation of DNA replication).

On the basis of a single muscle sample for DNA content determinations (22), total muscle nuclear population in normal male Sprague-Dawley rats is achieved by 8 weeks of age, with a spurt in DNA accumulation during puberty (6 to 8 weeks). In the female after 3 weeks of age the number of nuclei increase much more slowly than in the male. In addition, there is little acceleration during puberty, resulting in final nuclear numbers of approximately two-thirds of the male value at 14 weeks. The discrepancy between the figure of 90 to 95 days, cited earlier, and this value of 8 weeks or 56 days for the age of cessation of DNA growth in rat skeletal muscle may relate to the problems of extrapolation from a single specimen to total muscle DNA content.

Methods of assessing muscle cell growth in the human must be adapted to biopsy sampling for the biochemical measurements of DNA and protein. All the reservations we have noted about the reliability of a single sample for the assessment of DNA content of the entire skeletal musculature pertain to human studies as well as to rat data. Such biopsy data, however, are the only ones available for the human.

Creatinine excretion has been used to measure total muscle mass. Graystone (50) ably reviews the early studies that support the high correlation between the fat-free body mass and urinary creatinine levels. Under the conditions of a low creatinine, low hydroxyproline diet for three days before and including three consecutive days of urine collections (muscle mass in kilograms) equals (mean urinary creatinine excretion in grams per day times 20). The derivation of this factor of 20 is well documented in Graystone's paper. The relationships of creatinine excretion to body weight, height, age, and bone age for normal males and females are shown in Tables 2 and 3, respectively. Linear relationships with high coefficients of correlation are obtained in normal children with no apparent sex difference when creatinine excretion in milligrams per day is plotted against body weight. When height is used as a base-

## Table 2  Creatinine Excretion in Normal Boys: Relationship with Weight, Height, Chronologic Age, and Bone Age[a]

| | Equation | N | Correlation Coefficient | Standard Deviation (mg/24) |
|---|---|---|---|---|
| *Weight* | | | | |
| Infants (0.18–1.5 yr) | CREAT = 11.73 (WT) − 3.631 | 22 | 0.82 | 19 |
| Boys (5–16 yr) | CREAT = 24.263 (WT) − 149.624 | 19 | 0.94 | 113 |
| *Height* | | | | |
| Infants (0.18–1.5 yr) | CREAT = 3.183 (HT) − 130.927 | 22 | 0.86 | 16 |
| Boys (5–16 yr) | CREAT = 3288.506 − 55.213 (HT) + 0.257 (HT)$^2$ | 19 | | 90 |
| ≥137.5 cm | CREAT = 25.6 (HT) − 3027.7 | 12 | | 102 |
| ≤137.5 cm | CREAT = 6.4 (HT) − 383.9 | 7 | | 26 |
| *Chronologic age* | | | | |
| Infants (0.18–1.5 yr) | CREAT = 55.217 (CA) + 46.0 | 22 | 0.79 | 20 |
| Boys (5–16 yr) | CREAT = 650.019 − 105.493 (CA) + 9.516 (CA)$^2$ | 19 | | 103 |
| *Bone age* | | | | |
| Boys (5–16 yr) | CREAT = 90.24 (BA) − 149.81 | 17 | 0.95 | 100 |

[a] Reprinted from *Human Growth*, D. B. Cheek, Ed. Philadelphia: Lea & Febiger, 1968, p. 184.

**Table 3  Creatinine Excretion in Normal Girls: Relationship with Weight, Height, Chronologic Age, and Bone Age**[a]

|  | Equation | N | Correlation Coefficient | Standard Deviation (mg/24 hr) |
|---|---|---|---|---|
| Weight | CREAT = 20.901 (WT) − 75.394 | 20 | 0.915 | 109 |
| Height | CREAT = 12.784 (HT) − 1136.676 | 19 | 0.93 | 95 |
| Chronologic age | CREAT = 69.005 (CA) − 97.74 | 20 | 0.91 | 102 |
| Bone age | CREAT = 62.29 (BA) − 65.81 | 20 | 0.93 | 99 |
| Height and weight | CREAT = 8.8183 (HT) + 6.8694 (WT) − 821.0265 | 19 | 0.94 | 94 |

[a] Reprinted from *Human Growth*, D. B. Cheek, Ed. Philadelphia: Lea & Febiger, 1968, p. 184.

line, normal males and females have similar amounts of muscle per unit height until a height of 137.5 cm is reached. Thereafter growth in muscle mass in boys accelerates rapidly, achieving values at early adolescence of one and one-half to two times the values per unit height noted in normal females. Sex differences, especially in later childhood, occur when creatinine excretion is compared with chronological or bone age. Graystone (50) has also determined the mathematical relationships between creatinine excretion and total body water, extracellular volume, total body chloride, total body potassium, and intracellular water. This remarkable investigation documents normal growth in muscle mass in childhood and describes its relation to the other major body compartments. It provides valuable baseline information for the study of abnormal growth. However, if muscle mass calculations are to be made from creatinine excretion values in abnormal growth states, such as malnutrition, it will be important to determine whether Graystone's factor of 20 holds for the abnormal state as well.

Using a single muscle biopsy and 24-hour creatinine excretion, Cheek (20) calculated total muscle nuclear population from the equation [(DNA content per gram of muscle) divided by (DNA content per diploid nucleus)] times (total muscle mass in grams). He determined that muscle nuclear number in male infants increases linearly with age, length, total body water, and basal oxygen consumption. The equations are given in Table 4. No data are available for males between $1\frac{1}{2}$ and 5 years of age. From 5 to $10\frac{1}{2}$ years the mathematical relationship between muscle nuclear number and age is again linear. The slope of the line, however, is less; that is, the rate of DNA replication in muscle tissue is less rapid in the older boys. At the age of $10\frac{1}{2}$ years the rate of DNA replication in muscle tissue again accelerates (Fig. 4). From 5 to 16 years growth in muscle nuclear number is linear with total

**Table 4  Muscle Nuclear Number in Male Infants of 0.18 to 1.5 Years of Age**[a]

| Nuclear Number $\times 10^{12}$ | N | Coefficient Correlation | SD |
|---|---|---|---|
| Number = 0.0895 (CA) + 0.206 | 17 | 0.66 | 0.043 |
| = 0.00503 (HT) − 0.076 | 17 | 0.73 | 0.0396 |
| = 0.02915 (TW) + 0.116 | 14 | 0.70 | 0.043 |
| = 0.0076  (Cals/hr) + 0.118 | 13 | 0.93 | 0.025 |

[a] Adapted from *Human Growth*, D. B. Cheek, Ed. Philadelphia: Lea & Febiger, 1968.
CA: chronologic age in years.
HT: height in centimeters.
TW: total body water in liters.

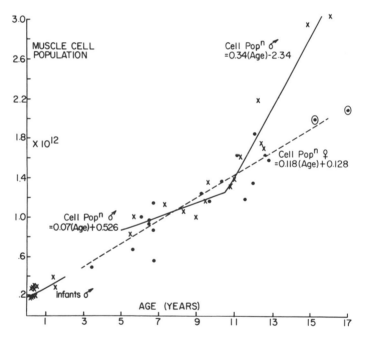

**Fig. 4.** Muscle nuclear number in children versus age for normal children. X's represent individual points of data for males. The dots represent individual points of data for females. The equations for the separate lines are recorded. Reprinted from *Human Growth*, D. B. Cheek, ed. Philadelphia: Lea & Febiger, 1968, p. 340.

body water and basal oxygen consumption. The equations for these relationships are listed in Table 5. Estimates of the number of muscle nuclei in males at various ages follow:

| Age | Nuclear Number |
| --- | --- |
| 2 months | $0.22 \times 10^{12}$ |
| 1.5 years | $0.34 \times 10^{12}$ |
| 5 years | $0.90 \times 10^{12}$ |
| 10 years | $1.22 \times 10^{12}$ |
| 16 years | $3.10 \times 10^{12}$ |

These results represent an overall 14-fold increase in nuclear number from 2 months to 16 years of age.

In normal females from 6 to 17 years growth in muscle nuclear number is linear with age, but in contrast to males there is no acceleration in the rate of DNA replication during adolescence (Fig. 4). Muscle nuclear number is also linear with height, total body water, and basal oxygen consumption (Table 5). There are sex differences with age and height but not with total body water or basal oxygen consumption. The equation for the relation between total body water and muscle nuclear number for both sexes combined is also given in Table 6.

Using the protein/DNA ratio, Cheek (20) has followed growth in "cell mass" in normal children. When this ratio is related to an indicator of lean body mass such as total body water, a definite sex difference is noted (Fig. 5). During the midchildhood years females have a larger "cell mass" than males.

Cell mass reaches stable, presumably adult levels at a total body water value of 20.3 l, which is equivalent to the age of $10\frac{1}{2}$ years in the normally growing female. The end point for cell mass in males is not defined. Cell mass, however, continues to increase in males to at least 16 years of age. By $4\frac{1}{2}$ years of age (total body water of 30 l) male values equal female values and thereafter exceed them.

Although these extensive studies of Dr. Cheek and his coworkers depend on assumptions of constancy of DNA content and constancy of ratios of fiber to nonfiber nuclei in all skeletal muscle and at all ages from birth to adolescence, their importance to our understanding of cellular growth in human muscle cannot be overstated. The validity of the assumptions remains to be substantiated and the numerical results may change with further studies. The trends described in cell growth with maturation and development cannot, however, be expected to

**Table 5  Muscle Nuclear Number in Older Children**[a]

| Nuclear Number $\times 10^{12}$ | N | Coefficient Correlation | SD |
|---|---|---|---|
| *Males* | | | |
| Number = 0.0706 (CA) + 0.526 | 7 | | 0.171 |
|     if CA $\leq$ 10.5 years | | | |
|     = 0.0342 (CA) − 2.34 | 8 | | 0.171 |
|     if CA $\geq$ 10.5 years | | | |
|     = 0.0877 (TW) − 0.329 | 15 | 0.92 | 0.27 |
|     = 0.0466 (Cals/hr) − 0.683[b] | 15 | 0.70 | 0.51 |
| *Females* | | | |
| Number = 0.118 (CA) + 0.128 | 19 | 0.93 | 0.173 |
|     = 0.021 (HT) − 1.492 | 19 | 0.91 | 0.191 |
|     = 0.0646 (TW) − 0.085 | 19 | 0.89 | 0.212 |
|     = 0.0577 (Cals/hr) − 1.208[b] | 19 | 0.84 | 0.27 |
| *Males and Females* | | | |
| Number = 0.0807 (TW) − 0.1634 | 29 | 0.97 | 0.205 |

[a] Adapted from *Human Growth*, D. B. Cheek, Ed. Philadelphia: Lea & Febiger, 1968.
[b] No sex difference.
CA: chronologic age in years.
HT: height in centimeters.
TW: total body water in liters.

**Table 6  Incorporation of $^{14}$C-Thymidine into DNA**[a]

| | | |
|---|---|---|
| 16 days | 400 (300–480) | 130 (90–180) |
| 18 days | 18 (16–20) | 550 (480–600) |
| 20 days | 18 (16–20) | 600 (520–630) |
| Background | 18 (16–20) | 18 (16–20) |

Figures expressed as cpm/mg DNA. Each figure represents the average of 10 placentas or embryos. Figures in parentheses represent range.

[a] Reprinted from *Nature* **212,** 34 (1966).

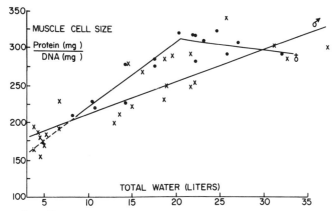

**Fig. 5.** Muscle cell size (protein/DNA ratio) versus total body water in normal children. X's represent individual points of data for males; the dots represent individual points of data for females. Reprinted from *Human Growth*, D. B. Cheek, Ed., Philadelphia: Lea & Febiger, 1968, p. 345.

change significantly and therein lies their import. This group has used the only techniques currently available for the study of human growth and has provided a wealth of data that can be altered or changed only with the advance of technology.

## Placenta

Since placenta is readily available for study, abnormalities in fetal growth that are paralleled in the placenta could more easily be investigated by using placenta. With this in mind, placental growth has been examined in the normal rat and human and under certain abnormal conditions known to affect the growth of the fetus.

Using radioautography, Jollie has demonstrated that labeled mitotic figures do not appear in the trophoblastic layer of rat placenta after the eighteenth day of gestation (63). Our own studies demonstrate that although weight, protein, and RNA rise linearly until the twentieth day DNA fails to increase after the seventeenth day owing to a cessation of DNA synthesis (113). Table 6 demonstrates a failure of incorporation of $^{14}$C thymidine into placental DNA between the sixteenth and eighteenth day. Hence cell division stops around the seventeenth day and the rest of the growth is due to an increase in protoplasmic elements without further cell division. Thus three phases of cellular growth may be described in rat placenta just as in the other organs of the rat. From the tenth day until about the sixteenth day of gestation DNA synthesis and net protein synthesis are proportional and cell number increases, whereas cell size is unchanged. This is the period of pure hyperplasia. From the sixteenth to the eighteenth day, as a consequence of a slowing in the rate of DNA synthesis with protein synthesis continuing at the same rate, hyperplasia and hypertrophy are occurring together. Finally, around the eighteenth day cell division stops altogether. Weight and protein still continue their linear rise. The ratios rapidly increase. Hypertrophy is occurring alone (Fig. 6).

PLACENTAL GROWTH

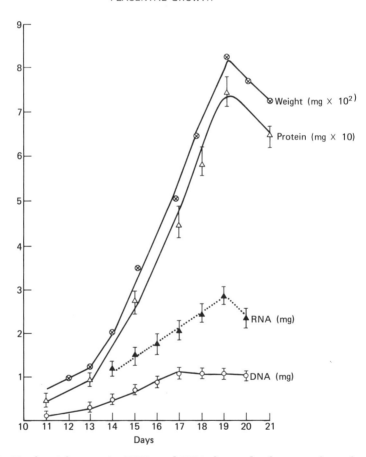

Fig. 6. Total weight, protein, DNA, and RNA during development of rat placenta. Each point represents the average of at least 15 separate determinations. The bars on the figure represent the range. Reprinted from *Nature* **212**, 34 (1966).

Maturational changes occur throughout gestation. Therefore growth by cell division is not necessary for certain of these maturational changes to occur. During the final period of hypertrophy certain electronmicroscopic changes take place in the rat placenta. There is a reduction of the "placental barrier" with the appearance of endothelial and trophoblastic fenestrations. Increased micropinocytotic 'activity, irregularities at the inner plasma membrane, and the appearance of large vacuoles can all be seen in the so-called element III. There is also approximation of inner and outer membranes at points of constriction and formation of pediclelike foot processes (63).

Concomitant with these morphologic changes, profound functional changes take place. There is a change in the selectivity of transportable materials and an increase in the transport rate of certain materials. Also, glycogen, which had previously been deposited in copious amounts, rapidly becomes depleted (26).

Although the exact timing of events is not so clear as with rats, available data indicate that human placenta grows in a qualitatively similar manner. Placenta is the only human tissue in which cellular growth has been studied throughout its entire life-span. Therefore it is not known whether the sequence to be described is characteristic of other human tissues. Studies cited in the preceding section would indicate, however, that human brain grows in a qualitatively similar manner.

Our data (108), which show a linear relationship between placental and fetal weight, agree with the data of previous investigators. We have not studied enough cases of more than 3500 g to exclude a terminal falling off in the rate of placental growth as suggested by Gruenwald and Minn (52), but, at least until the fetus reaches 3500 g, fetal weight gain is accompanied by a linear increase in the weight of the placenta. It has also been shown that both total protein and RNA increase linearly to term. DNA, however, ceases to increase after the placenta reaches about 300 g (Fig. 7). This corresponds to a fetal weight of about 2400 g or a gestational age of 34 to 36 weeks. Thus, as demonstrated in the rat, cell division ceases before term. In the human this appears to be about the thirty-fifth week of gestation.

Data of Beaconsfield et al. (10) suggest that this cessation of DNA synthesis is accompanied by a shift in the pathway of glucose metabolism away from the hexosemonophosphate shunt, hence away from nucleic acid synthesis.

Although the cellular events are similar during the growth of human and rat placenta, there is one quantitative difference. The RNA/DNA ratio is twice as high in the rat. The reason for this difference is unknown, but it may be due to increased connective tissue within the

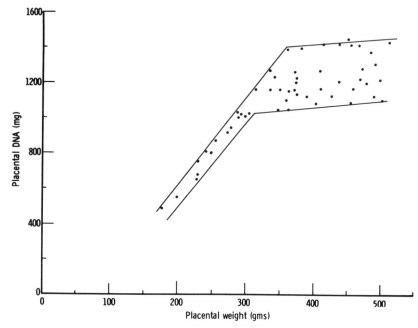

Fig. 7.   Placental DNA versus fetal weight. Reprinted from *Pediatrics* **39,** 250 (1967).

human placenta. Fibroblasts contain relatively little RNA. Possibly the trophoblasts contain equal quantities of RNA in both species.

Maturation in human placenta also occurs throughout all three growth periods (53). Again, cell division is not essential to differentiation, either morphologically or functionally, but, although growth in the two species proceeds for the most part in a similar fashion, differentiation, at least in certain biochemical areas, may be quite different. Although both rat and human placenta lose glycogen as term approaches, there are differences in carbohydrate metabolism, at least in vitro.

Ginsberg et al. (45) have demonstrated that lactic acid production in vitro is much greater in rat than in human placenta. Furthermore, adrenaline does not increase lactate production in rat placenta as it does in human. Similarly, glucose uptake is greater in rat placenta and is not enhanced by either anaerobiosis or the addition of adrenaline. Placental glycogen breakdown during incubation is much greater in rat than in human and is not influenced in the rat by adding adrenaline. In summary, then, normal cellular growth of placenta proceeds through an orderly sequence of changes as gestation progresses. Therefore the time at which a stimulus is exerted may be as important as the nature of the stimulus itself. The same stimulus acting early might interfere with cell division, whereas later it cannot. Conversely, the nature of the cellular effects produced might give a clue to the time an unknown stimulus was most active. In any event, the DNA, RNA, and protein content of the placenta can be examined under conditions known to affect both fetal and placental growth. The similarity in the growth pattern between rat and human placenta also suggests the possibility of using the rat as an experimental model.

## NUTRITIONAL EFFECTS ON CELLULAR GROWTH

The environmental condition that has been most extensively studied during early development is nutrition. The commonest method employed in altering the nutritional status of neonatal rats is to vary the number of pups nursing from a single mother. The normal rat litter consists of 8 to 12 pups and therefore a nursing group of 10 animals has arbitrarily been considered normal. Malnutrition is imposed by increasing the size of the nursing group to 18 animals and overnutrition by decreasing the size to three.

More recently other methods of undernutrition have been employed. Protein restriction in the lactating mother reduces the quantity of milk produced without altering its composition. Allowing the animals to nurse for only a single eight-hour period per day also reduces the quantity of milk consumed. All these methods produce a total caloric restriction as well as a restriction in individual nutrients, the most notable of which is protein. So far all three methods have produced comparable results on brain growth, and therefore we shall examine them together.

In order to produce qualitative changes in the milk without changing the quantity produced the nursing animal must be artificially fed. The two procedures that have been employed are repeated tube feeding and gastrostomy with continuous infusion of liquid. Both are time consuming, extremely tedious, and technically difficult. At present there are no data on cellular growth of the brain based on these feeding techniques, although Miller has used repeated tube feeding extensively to study protein synthesis in the developing liver (74).

Employing the "large and small litter" technique, McCance and Widdowson (97) demonstrated a number of years ago that the growth rate of the nursing pups was inversely proportional to the number of animals in the group. Moreover, they demonstrated that the weight of the brain was reduced in the undernourished animals and increased in the overnourished animals. Perhaps the most important finding in these experiments was that no matter what the state of nutrition after weaning the undernourished animals never attained normal size and their brains never recovered normal weight. Other experiments with neonatal pigs confirmed these results. Profound growth retardation in the pigs was produced in the neonatal period and complete recovery in either body size or brain size could not be obtained even when maximum nutritional rehabilitation was attempted (31).

Previous studies had indicated that undernutrition later in the growing period of the rat would retard growth, but that nutritional rehabilitation could restore normal body weight and brain weight (61). The factor that determined whether the animal recovered appeared to be the time at which malnutrition occurred. The earlier the undernutrition, the less likely the recovery after the stimulus was discontinued. Thus early growth differs from later growth in some way that allows the older animal to recover from malnutrition.

## Brain

The studies of normal cellular growth outlined above suggest a possible explanation. Early organ growth is mainly due to cell division and an increase in the number of cells. Later organ growth is due to hypertrophy with already present individual cells becoming larger. When the original McCance and Widdowson experiments were repeated and compared with data from animals undernourished at two later times during the growing period, it became clear that if malnutrition were imposed during the proliferative phase of growth the rate of cell division was slowed and the ultimate number of cells was reduced. Moreover, this change was permanent and could not be reversed once the normal time for cell division had passed (112). In contrast, undernutrition imposed during the period when cells are normally enlarging will curtail the enlargement, but on subsequent rehabilitation the cells will resume their normal size. These experiments demonstrated that total brain cell number could be permanently reduced by undernourishing the rat during the first 21 days of life and that no matter what feeding regimen was attempted thereafter this reduction in cell number would persist (112).

If the reduction in brain size in the animals reared in litters of 18 was due to a reduced number of cells, what about those animals reared in litters of three? When these experiments were performed, it became clear that the overnourished animals had an increased number of brain cells when compared with animals nursed in normal-sized litters (114). Hence the number of cells attained by the developing rat brain depends, in part, on the nutrition of the animal during the time when brain cells are undergoing active proliferation. Subsequent experiments have demonstrated that the rate of cell division can actually be manipulated in either direction by changing the state of nutrition during the proliferative phase (109). Thus undernutrition for the first nine days of life produces a deficit in brain-cell number which can be entirely overcome by overnourishing the animal for the next 12 days. Note that we cannot differentiate one cell type from another with these methods. It is therefore possible that the deficit is made up by the proliferation of a different type of cell than was inhibited during the earlier restriction.

Malnutrition in rats during the first three weeks of life has been shown to interfere with the synthesis of lipids (27, 29, 30). There is a substantial deficit in total brain cholesterol and a lowering of cholesterol concentration. In pigs malnourished during the first year of life total brain cholesterol and phospholipid content are markedly reduced and cholesterol concentration is slightly reduced (31). These changes, both in rats and in pigs, persist even when the animals are rehabilitated for a long time. More recently, it has been demonstrated that the incorporation of sulfatide into myelin of rat brain is reduced both in vivo and in vitro by malnutrition during the first three weeks of life. Moreover, the activity of galactocerebroside sulfokinase, the enzyme responsible for this incorporation, is reduced during malnutrition (19). Although the reduced lipid content could be due to a reduction in the number of oligodendroglia, the enzymatic data suggest that lipid synthesis per cell may also be reduced.

Examining myelination by measuring lipid deposition gives us two types of data: lipid concentration and total lipid content. The increase in lipid concentration, which is mainly due to a reduction in water content, represents a progressive increase in sheath thickness and has therefore been regarded as a "maturity index." In contrast, the increase in total lipid content represents the growth in length or number of axons and either the elongation of existing myelin sheaths or the laying down of new ones. Thus malnutrition before weaning in the rat results not only in fewer or shorter sheaths, as assessed by reduced total brain cholesterol, but also in thinner myelin sheaths, since the concentration of cholesterol is also reduced. In the pig, by contrast, although the number or length of the sheaths is reduced, the thickness would appear to be nearly normal, since there is little effect on cholesterol concentration.

Regional patterns of cellular growth are also modified by malnutrition during the nursing period (43). Cerebellum, in which the rate of cell division is most rapid, is affected earliest (by eight days of life) and most markedly. Cerebrum, in which cell division is occurring at a slower rate, is affected later (at 14 days of life) and less markedly (Fig. 8). The effects produced include a reduced rate of cell division in both areas as well as a reduction in overall protein synthesis and in the synthesis of various lipids. In addition to these effects on areas of rapid

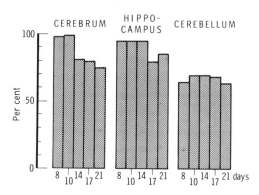

Fig. 8. Effect of neonatal caloric restriction on total DNA content of various brain regions. Reprinted from *Fed. Proc.* **29**, 1512 (1970).

cell division, the increase in DNA content, which normally appears in hippocampus between the fourteenth and seventeenth day, is delayed and perhaps even partly prevented (Fig. 8). It would appear from these data that those regions in which the rate of cell division is highest are affected earliest and most markedly and that cell migration is also curtailed. Whether this is actually an interference with migratory patterns or an inhibition of cell division at the source below the lateral ventricle is not fully known, but data to be discussed shortly strongly suggest that the latter accounts for at least some of the reduced cell number in hippocampus. Regional patterns of lipid synthesis and the effects of malnutrition on these patterns have not been clearly established. The available data, however, suggest that areas in which myelination is most rapid are most vulnerable to the effects of early malnutrition.

This raises an interesting question that has not yet been investigated. Although the reduction in lipid content and the reduction in DNA content are proportional in whole brain so that the lipid/DNA ratio is unchanged, our previous interpretation of a normal lipid content per cell may not be reflecting a true pattern for individual regions. It may be applicable only to the "average cell." It is conceivable that the reduction in DNA content in a region with little lipid synthesis is matched by a reduction in lipid content in a region in which DNA synthesis has already slowed down or stopped. Under these conditions the first region would contain fewer cells but the second would have reduced lipid content per cell. The actual effect of malnutrition in the area involved in lipid synthesis would be to lower the amount of lipid per cell, but this effect would be masked when both regions were studied together. For this reason it is important that regional studies of the effect of malnutrition on lipid synthesis in brain be undertaken and correlated with regional studies of DNA synthesis in the same brains. Regional studies of the various enzymes controlling the rate of cell division and the effects of malnutrition on these enzymes are just beginning, and it is too early to draw any conclusions. There have been no regional studies yet of the enzymes involved in lipid synthesis, the pathway of glucose metabolism, or the effect of malnutrition on these parameters. Recent data have indicated that malnutrition will elevate cytoplasmic RNAse activity in young rat brain and that this is due largely to a diminution in activity of the RNAse inhibitor protein.[*] More studies of this type are needed in whole brain and various brain regions to obtain a more complete picture of the effects of malnutrition on the cellular and chemical growth of the brain.

In all of the discussion to this point individual cell types have not been considered. Up to now, three types of study have been conducted on the brains of animals malnourished during rapid growth. The first is careful histologic examination in which a variety of special stains is employed. The second is histochemical examination in an attempt to differentiate effects on patterns of specific enzyme development. The third is radioautographic studies to determine the effect of undernutrition on the division of particular cell types. Unfortunately the same species have not been employed in all these studies, which makes cross comparisons very difficult.

Histologic changes have been observed in the central nervous systems of rats, pigs, and dogs reared after weaning on protein-deficient diets (76, 77). Both neurones and glia in spinal cord and medulla degenerate. These changes persist even after intensive rehabilitation with a protein-rich diet lasting for as long as three months. The changes could be made more severe either by beginning the restriction at an earlier age or by extending the duration of the deficient diet. In pigs it has also been demonstrated that severe undernutrition early in life produces histologic changes in the cortex itself. Neurones in the gray matter are reduced in number and appear to be swollen. More recently histochemical changes have been described in the brains of rats submitted to early

[*] P. Rosso, M. Nelson, and M. Winick, unpublished data.

malnutrition (120). The appearance of a variety of enzymes, demonstrable by special staining techniques, is delayed and the ultimate quantity obtained is reduced. Thus early malnutrition produces specific histologic and histochemical changes within the cells of the central nervous system. Again, the earlier the malnutrition, the more severe the damage and the more likely it is to persist.

Radioautographic studies in our laboratory indicate that in neonatal rats malnourished for the first 10 days of life only glial cell division is inhibited in cerebrum, since neuronal cell division ceases before birth. In cerebellum the rate of cell division of external granular cells, internal granular cells, and molecular cells is reduced. In addition, the rate of cell division in neurones under the third and lateral ventricles is decreased (Fig. 9). This reduction in neurones under the lateral ventricle

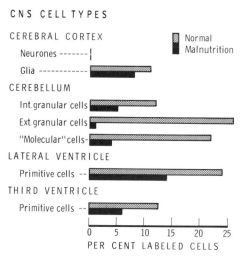

Fig. 9. Effect of maternal protein restriction on various cell types in fetal brain. Reprinted from *Fed. Proc.* **29**, 1513 (1970).

explains, at least in part, the reduced DNA content in hippocampus five days later, since these are the cells that are destined to migrate into the hippocampus.

Studies of the effects of malnutrition on cellular growth of human brain have been quite limited. The data indicate that in marasmic infants who died of malnutrition during the first year of life wet weight, dry weight, total protein, total RNA, total cholesterol (Fig. 10) total phospholipid, and total DNA (Fig. 11) content are proportionally reduced (29, 115). Thus the rate of DNA synthesis is slowed, cell division is

TOTAL HUMAN BRAIN CHOLESTEROL

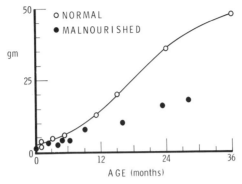

**Fig. 10.** Total cholesterol content of human brain at various ages. Adapted from *Amer. J. Clin. Nutr.* **23**, 1278, (1970).

curtailed, and the result is a reduced number of cells. Since the reduction in the other elements is proportional to the reduction in DNA content, the ratios are unchanged, hence the size of cells or the lipid content per cell is not altered. Again it is to be emphasized that these are "average" cells we are describing, and it is quite possible that certain cells (i.e., those with lipid being actively deposited) are being affected differently from those in which this deposition is not occurring. If the malnutrition persists beyond about 8 months of age, not only is the number

NUMBER OF CELLS IN HUMAN BRAIN

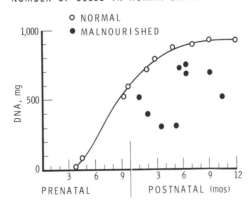

**Fig. 11.** Line indicates normal mean for U.S. population, ○ indicates normal Chilean children, ● indicates Chilean children who died of severe malnutrition during the first year of life. Reprinted from *Pediat. Res.* **3**, 183 (1969).

of cells reduced but also the size of individual cells. In addition, the lipid per cell is reduced (Fig. 12). Thus in human brain there is a similar type of response to malnutrition. During proliferative growth cell division is curtailed; during hypertrophic growth the normal enlargement in cells is prevented.

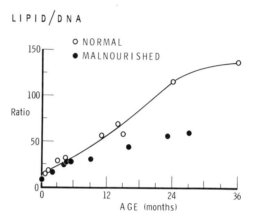

LIPID/DNA

Fig. 12.  Lipid-DNA ratio in normal and malnourished children at different ages. Reprinted from *Amer J. Clin. Nutr.* 23, 1278 (1970).

If we interpret the lipid data as previously discussed, myelination in the human brain would be affected in a manner more analogous to the pig brain than to the rat brain. Total cholesterol or phospholipid content is reduced; hence the number or length of myelin sheaths is also reduced. Both phospholipid concentration and cholesterol concentration are unaffected, however. Hence the thickness of those myelin sheaths that are present is unaffected. We could therefore argue that the major effect of malnutrition is to interfere with cellular growth. During the first eight months of life this interference reduces the number of glia, specifically oligodendroglia, and myelination is proportionally reduced. Continued malnutrition reduces cell size. In neurones this would probably be associated with a reduction in the number or length of processes. Again myelination is proportionally curtailed. However, the deposition of myelin around those processes that are present and do grow proceeds normally, and the thickness of the myelin sheath is normal, since the concentration of cholesterol and phospholipids remains unchanged. Note that this interpretation is based on only limited observations and therefore more data must be collected. For the present this appears to be a reasonable working hypothesis.

Thus postnatal malnutrition will affect cell division and myelination in the developing rat and human brain. In both it would appear that the vulnerable periods coincide with the maximum rate of synthesis of DNA and myelin. All regions seem to be vulnerable, but the timing of their vulnerability will vary, again depending on the maximum rate of synthesis in the particular region. All cell types so far studied are affected if they are dividing at the time the undernutrition occurs. In the rat recovery appears to be possible only if the nutritional status is changed during these vulnerable periods.

## Muscle

During hyperplastic growth in the rat protein-calorie malnutrition will result in a retardation in the rate of DNA synthesis in gastrocnemius muscle (112). There is little change in the protein/DNA ratio, and the number of nuclei remain reduced even after adequate refeeding. Malnutrition in the more mature postpubertal animal (112) results in a reduced protein/DNA ratio only, and this change is reversed with refeeding.

In muscle of young rats fed a diet low in both calories and protein, Hill et al. (56) have found a marked reduction in both DNA content and protein/DNA ratio. By contrast, when the animals were restricted in calories but were fed adequate protein, less reduction in muscle growth or muscle nuclear number was noted. In these animals the protein/DNA ratios were either normal or slightly increased. These authors postulate that reducing caloric intake will affect DNA replication primarily, but the reduction of caloric and protein intake has more serious effects on intracellular protein synthesis as well.

In laboratory studies of malnutrition we can control the diet the animals receive and can usually produce a specific type of malnutrition. In clinical studies, however, patients rarely exhibit pure marasmus or pure kwashiorkor but present a picture of mixed protein-calorie malnutrition. In the literature on muscle growth in human malnutrition the age of onset, duration of malnutrition, severity of malnutrition, and type of dietary deficiency are variable; hence it is difficult to generalize regarding effects on cellular growth of muscle. It seems clear, however, that whether estimated from cadaver analysis (92), biopsy specimen (93), limb measurements (83), or creatinine excretion (2, 23, 83), muscle growth is more severely and disproportionately reduced than the reduction in total body weight alone would indicate. Loss of total body potassium (2) and muscle tissue protein (92, 93) can often be severe. Concomitantly, there is an increase in total body water (2, 49) when compared with body weight which is primarily due to expansion of the extracellular fluid compartment.

In a study of nine male Peruvian infants, 5 to 30 months of age and suffering from severe malnutrition (23), gluteal muscle samples were analyzed for DNA and protein content and creatinine excretion was used to assess muscle mass. The most striking change was a reduction of the protein/DNA ratio, which indicated a loss of "cell mass." There was only a slight reduction in muscle nuclear number when compared with infants of a similar height. These data conflict with data cited elsewhere in this review which have demonstrated decreased DNA content in other tissues with severe infantile malnutrition. There are several possible explanations for this discrepancy. First, the calculation of nuclear number depends on the DNA concentration of the biopsy specimen, which may not reflect DNA content in muscles throughout the body. Second, the calculation depends on the assumption that the factor for conversion of creatinine excretion to muscle mass is the same in normal and malnourished children. This has not been entirely substantiated; indeed Alleyne's work (2) suggests that the factor of 20 may be in error for malnourished children. Finally, DNA replication and cell division are time-related phenomena and are logically better compared with controls of the same chronological age rather than the same height, as done in this study. Since these Peruvian children were retarded in growth, we might expect reductions in nuclear number if the comparisons were made against an age baseline. Until further studies substantiate the validity of the factor of 20 for creatinine excretion conversion or until the DNA content of an entire muscle is measured, we must conclude that the extent of the effects of infantile malnutrition on muscle nuclear number have not yet been precisely delineated.

### Placenta and Fetus

During intrauterine life all organs of the fetus are in the hyperplastic phase of growth. At no other time should the organism be more susceptible to nutritional stresses, yet only recently has any information about fetal malnutrition been forthcoming. This is true probably for two reasons, one operational and the other philosophical. The first was the relative inaccessibility of the fetus for experimental manipulation. The second has been the generally accepted view of the fetus as the perfect parasite, extracting its needs from its mother. Recently, as researchers have ventured into the uterus, this widely accepted viewpoint is being challenged. Fetal malnutrition may result from reduced maternal circulation, inadequate nutrients within the maternal circulation, or faulty placental transport of specific nutrients. The first two situations are now being extensively investigated in experimental animals.

The supply of blood to a single fetus in an animal delivering a litter of fetuses may be reduced spontaneously. It is not uncommon to see a "runt" in a litter of dogs or cats, and it is common knowledge that these animals will survive only with special care and that they will never reach the same final size as their littermates even if this special care is given. Occasionally the same situation occurs in a litter of pigs. Widdowson has studied the cellular changes that take place in the organs of these spontaneously occurring "runt" pigs. Her findings indicate that cell division has been curtailed in heart, kidney, brain, and skeletal muscle, the only organs studied so far. Cell size was also reduced in all organs studied when compared with littermate controls (96).

Blood supply in the rat can be artificially reduced by clamping the uterine artery supplying one uterine horn. Using this technique, Wiggleworth (99) compared the growth of the fetuses in the ligated horn to that of the fetuses in the unligated horn. Growth rate was reduced proportionally to the distance of the particular fetus from the ligated artery. Those at the uterine end closest to the ligation generally died. As one progressed farther away from the ligated uterine artery and closer to the intact ovarian artery, growth rate increased. More recently the cellular growth of various fetal organs, including placenta, has been studied in surviving animals within the ligated horn. Ligation on the thirteenth day of gestation will affect the rate of cell division in both placenta and other fetal organs. Ligation on the seventeenth day will again curtail cell division in the fetal organs, but in the placenta cell size will be reduced and cell number will remain normal (102). Thus in currently available animal studies in which blood supply has been artificially or spontaneously curtailed the rate of cell division in fetal organs has been retarded. Placenta, moreover, responds in a manner that might have been predicted from the earlier studies involving early postnatal malnutrition. Ligation during the period of hyperplasia results in reduced cell number, whereas ligation during hypertrophy results in reduced cell size. Therefore by determining the final effect on placental growth at delivery it may be possible to pinpoint the time at which a stimulus producing such a result must have been active. As we shall see, this possibility may have relevance in the human, in whom placenta is the only tissue readily available for study. Another abnormality was defined in placentas from the ligated horns—elevation of total organ RNA content, hence an elevation of the RNA/DNA ratio or RNA per cell (102). Such elevations in tissue RNA/DNA ratio have been described in several tissues under a variety of circumstances.

Clamping the aorta results in an increased RNA/DNA ratio in the left ventricle (47). Repeated nerve stimulation results in an elevation of the RNA/DNA ratio in the innervated muscle (70), injection of estrogen results in an increased RNA/DNA ratio in the uterus, and removal of one kidney will result in an increased RNA/DNA ratio in the contralateral kidney (64). The exact significance of this change is unknown, but it has been described under conditions requiring increased protein synthesis. This increase in placental RNA/DNA ratio may therefore represent an abortive attempt by placental cells to increase their rate of protein synthesis secondary to the stress of vascular insufficiency.

Maternal protein restriction in rats will also retard both placental and fetal growth. Cell number (DNA content) in placenta was reduced by 13 days after conception, cell size (protein/DNA ratio) remained normal, and the RNA/DNA ratio was markedly elevated (Table 7).

### Table 7    Effect of Maternal Malnutrition on Placenta[a]

|            | Control | Experimental |
|------------|---------|--------------|
| Weight     | .405    | .320         |
| Protein    | 28.0    | 21.7         |
| RNA        | 1.00    | 1.80         |
| DNA        | 1.06    | 0.82         |
| RNA/DNA    | 0.99    | 2.1          |
| Prot/DNA   | 27.0    | 28.2         |

[a] Data expressed in Mg. per whole placenta. Reprinted from *Diagnosis and Treatment of Fetal Disorders*, Karlis Adamsons, Ed. New York: Springer, 1969.

Retardation in fetal growth first became apparent at 15 days. After this there was a progressive decrease in cell number in all the organs studied (Table 8). By term there were only about 85% of the number of brain cells in control animals (102). These data agree with previous data of Zamenhof (119), which showed a similar reduction in total brain cell number in term fetuses whose mothers were exposed to a slightly different type of nutritional deprivation. Thus the cellular changes produced by severe prenatal food restriction are reflected in the placenta even earlier than in the fetus, but retardation of cell division in all fetal organs, including brain, can be clearly demonstrated.

### Table 8  Effect of Maternal Malnutrition on Fetal Tissues[a]

| Tissue | Percent Normal Control | | | |
| | Weight | Protein | RNA | DNA |
| --- | --- | --- | --- | --- |
| Whole animal | 87 | 81 | 83 | 81 |
| Brain | 91 | 85 | 82 | 84 |
| Heart | 84 | 84 | 79 | 81 |
| Lung | 82 | 85 | 85 | 89 |
| Liver | 82 | 80 | 85 | 85 |
| Kidney | 84 | 81 | 82 | 85 |

[a] Reprinted from *Diagnosis and Treatment of Fetal Disorders*, Karlis Adamsons, Ed. New York: Springer, 1969.

By employing radioautography after injecting the mother with tritiated thymidine cell division can be assessed in various discrete brain regions (Fig. 13). Differential regional sensitivity can be demonstrated in this

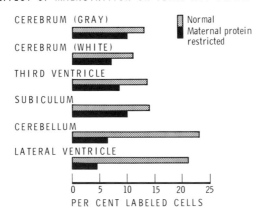

Fig. 13.  Effect of maternal protein restriction on regional DNA content of fetal brain. Reprinted from *Fed. Proc.* 29, 1513 (1970).

way by the sixteenth day of gestation in the brains of fetuses of protein-restricted mothers. The cerebral white and gray matter are mildly affected. The area adjacent to the third ventricle and the subiculum are moderately affected, whereas the cerebellum and the area directly adjacent to the lateral ventricle are markedly affected (107, 118). These data again demonstrate that the magnitude of the effect produced on cell division is directly related to the actual rate of cell division at the time the stimulus is applied. Moreover, they demonstrate that the maternal-placental barrier in the rat is not effective in protecting the fetal brain from discrete cellular effects caused by maternal food restriction.

The subsequent course of these animals born of protein-restricted mothers can be examined. Chow has reported that even if these animals are raised normally on foster mothers they demonstrate a permanent impairment in their ability to utilize nitrogen (68). Data from our own laboratory demonstrate that if these animals are nursed on normal foster mothers in normal-sized litters they will remain with a deficit in total brain cell number at weaning (107). Thus we can again see early programming of the ultimate number of brain cells. This program, moreover, is written in utero in response to maternal nutrition.

These same newborn pups of protein-restricted mothers may be subjected to postnatal nutritional manipulation. If they are raised in litters of three on normal foster mothers until weaning, the deficit in total number of brain cells may be almost entirely reversed (107). Although quantitatively the number of cells approaches normal, qualitatively the deficit at birth might very well be made up by an increase in cell number in different areas from those most affected in utero. Thus, although it may appear that optimally nourishing pups after exposing them to prenatal undernutrition will reverse the cellular effects, this may not actually be so in specific brain areas.

Perhaps the most analogous situation to the situation in humans is exposing these pups, malnourished in utero, to subsequent postnatal deprivation. These animals can be raised on foster mothers in groups of 18. Animals so reared show a marked reduction in brain cell number by weaning. This effect is much more pronounced than the effect of either prenatal or postnatal undernutrition alone (105, 106, 109) (Fig. 14). Animals subjected to prenatal malnutrition alone, as previously described, show a 15% reduction in total brain cell number at birth. Animals subjected only to postnatal malnutrition show a similar 15 to 20% reduction in brain cell number at weaning. In contrast, these "doubly deprived" animals demonstrate a 60% reduction in total brain cell number by weaning. These data demonstrate that malnutrition applied constantly throughout the entire period of brain cell proliferation will result in a profound reduction in brain cell number, greater than the sum of effects produced during various parts of the proliferative phase. It would appear that the duration of malnutrition as well as the severity during

MALNUTRITION
TOTAL BRAIN CELL NUMBER

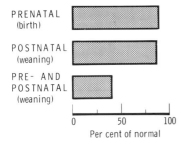

PRENATAL
(birth)

POSTNATAL
(weaning)

PRE- AND
POSTNATAL
(weaning)

0          50          100
Per cent of normal

Fig. 14. Comparison of caloric restriction after birth, protein restriction during gestation, and "combined" prenatal and postnatal restriction. Reprinted from *Fed. Proc* **29**, 1512 (1970).

this early critical period is extremely important in determining the ultimate cellular make-up of the brain (Fig. 14).

Recent experiments by Widdowson (96) in the guinea pig demonstrate that caloric restriction during gestation markedly reduces birth weight of the offspring and curtails the rate of cell division in the brain. In the skeletal muscle not only is there a reduction in cell number but the actual number of muscle fibers is reduced, and each muscle fiber has an increased number of nuclei. These animals when fed normally after birth fail to recover normal height or weight (96).

These animal data, then, clearly demonstrate that undernutrition due to reduced blood supply or reduced availability of nutrients will curtail placental and fetal growth, retard the rate of cell division in various fetal organs, and result in an animal whose organs contain fewer cells. Evidence also indicates that animals born after developing in this type of intrauterine environment will carry these cellular deficits for the rest of their lives.

Human placenta goes through the same three phases of growth as those described for the organs of the rat. Cell division ceases at about 34 to 36 weeks gestation, whereas weight and protein increase until nearly term (108).

Placentas from infants with "intrauterine growth failure" show fewer cells and an increased RNA/DNA ratio when compared with controls (101). Fifty percent of the placentas from an indigent population in Chile showed similar findings (106). Placentas from a malnourished population in Guatemala had fewer cells than normal.* In a single case of anorexia nervosa, in which a severely emaciated mother carried to term and gave birth to a 2500-g infant, the placenta contained less

* D. H. Dayton, L. J. Filer, and C. Conosa. Reported at 53rd annual Federation meeting, Atlantic City, New Jersey.

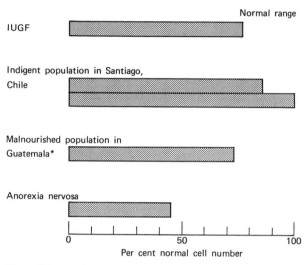

MALNUTRITION, HUMAN PLACENTA

**Fig. 15.** Placental cell number in various types of maternal undernutrition. Reprinted from *Clin. Obstet. Gynec.* 13, 537 (1970).

than 50% of the expected number of cells (106) (Fig. 15). Thus both vascular insufficiency and maternal malnutrition will curtail cell division in human placenta. The cellular make-up of the placenta in these situations strongly suggests that both stimuli have been active for some time before the thirty-fourth to thirty-sixth week of gestation.

The effects of those stimuli on the cellular growth of the fetus are more difficult to assess. Indirect evidence suggests that cell division in the human fetus may be retarded by maternal undernutrition. Fetal growth is retarded and birth weight reduced (85). If we examine available data on infants who died after exposure to severe postnatal malnutrition, three separate patterns emerge (Fig. 16). Breast-fed infants malnourished during the second year have a reduced protein/DNA ratio but a normal brain DNA content. Full-term infants who subsequently died of severe food deprivation during the first year of life had a 15 to 20% reduction in total brain cell number. Infants weighing 2000 g or less at birth who subsequently died of severe undernutrition during the first year of life showed a 60% reduction in total brain cell number (106). It is possible that these children were deprived *in utero* and represent a clinical counterpart of the "doubly deprived" animal. It is also possible that they were true premature infants and that the pre-

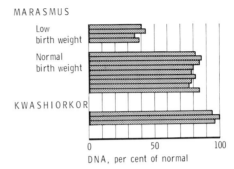

Fig. 16.  Total DNA content in brains of children who died of malnutrition. Reprinted from *Fed. Proc.* **29,** 1513 (1970).

mature is much more susceptible to postnatal malnutrition than the full-term infant.

## Other Tissues

The normal cellular growth patterns for most of the organs of the rat have been worked out. In general, weight and protein continue to increase until about 100 days of age. By contrast, DNA reaches a maximum before that in all organs. The time at which it does so varies with the particular organ (Fig. 17). In brain and lung DNA reaches a maximum at about 21 days of age, in liver, spleen, and kidney, at about

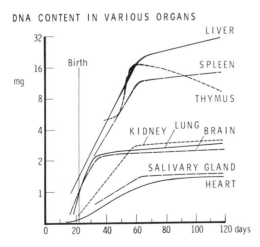

Fig. 17.  DNA milligrams during normal growth in the rat. Points represent mean values for at least 10 animals or organs. Reprinted from *Develop. Biol.* **23,** 454 (1970).

## Table 9  DNA Content of Various Organs in Normal Human Fetuses (milligrams)

| Weeks of gestation | 13 | 17 | 23 | 25 | 27 | 31 | 33 | 34 | 49 | 40 |
|---|---|---|---|---|---|---|---|---|---|---|
| Fetal weight (grams) | 31.7 | 163 | 320 | 580 | 610 | 1080 | 1525 | 1720 | 3300 | 4040 |
| Brain | 25 | 85 | 134 | 251 | 240 | 285 | 385 | — | 620 | 685 |
| Heart | 0.51 | 2.8 | 8.1 | 15.4 | 17.3 | 18.2 | 38.6 | 40.2 | 54.7 | 55.6 |
| Liver | 16.5 | 50 | 53.9 | 97.3 | 105.1 | 175 | 203 | 247 | 328 | 329 |
| Kidney | 0.72 | 6.8 | — | 38.7 | 59.6 | — | 73 | 79 | 107 | 128 |
| Spleen | 0.41 | 1.2 | 2.5 | 7.7 | 9.8 | 15.3 | — | 64.4 | 84.6 | 90.9 |
| Thyroid | 0.02 | 0.10 | — | 0.84 | 0.97 | 2.7 | — | 4.5 | 5.8 | 6.9 |
| Adrenal | 0.24 | 0.71 | 1.31 | 1.87 | 2.14 | 5.84 | 6.97 | 8.04 | 10.2 | 12.6 |
| Right lung | 3.0 | 23.6 | 50.9 | 64 | — | 66.4 | 68.5 | — | 148.7 | 166.8 |
| Left lung | 2.5 | 18.7 | 37.5 | 41.8 | — | 55.6 | 59.4 | — | 126 | 132 |
| Thymus | 0.39 | 3.99 | 10.96 | 21.8 | 26.5 | 47.3 | 105.4 | 160.6 | 249 | 303 |
| Esophagus | 0.17 | 0.60 | 0.64 | 0.78 | 0.80 | 1.38 | 3.69 | 4.21 | 6.1 | 6.9 |
| Stomach | 0.53 | 2.3 | 3.6 | 5.0 | 5.7 | 6.8 | 22.3 | 26.8 | 32.7 | 40.7 |
| Small intestine | 3.8 | 6.1 | 16.2 | 26.3 | 32.8 | 48.7 | 157 | 179 | 512 | 529 |
| Large intestine | 0.37 | 2.97 | 5.8 | 10.0 | 11.2 | 26.3 | 47.2 | 525 | 129.6 | 137.2 |
| Diaphragm | 0.38 | 2.1 | 5.2 | 6.8 | 7.2 | 18.7 | 24.7 | 31.7 | 385 | 45.3 |
| Tongue | 0.39 | 1.21 | 2.4 | 3.5 | 3.7 | 4.9 | — | — | — | — |

40 days, in submaxillary gland, at about 45 days, and in heart, at about 65 days. Malnutrition during the period of hyperplastic growth results in a reduced number of cells in all these organs.

In the human cellular growth patterns have been studied in 16 organs during normal fetal development. The data indicate that total cell number, as measured by total organ DNA content, increases in all organs from 13 weeks gestation until term. Cell size, as measured either by weight/DNA or protein/DNA ratios, remains unchanged throughout gestation in heart, kidney, spleen, thyroid, thymus, esophagus, stomach, large and small intestines, and tongue. In brain, lungs, liver, adrenal gland, and diaphragm cell size increases slowly from the beginning of the seventh month of gestation until term (Table 9).

More limited data during the first year of life demonstrate that cell number continues to increase rapidly in heart, liver, kidney, and spleen. Heart cell size begins to increase after three months of age, whereas in kidney, liver, and spleen cell size does not change during the first year (Table 10).

Table 10   DNA Content of Various Organs in Normal Infants

| Months after Birth | 2 | 3 | 5 | 10 | 12 |
|---|---|---|---|---|---|
| Weight | | | | | |
| Brain | — | 858 | 890 | 917 | 1000 |
| Heart | 72.8 | 88 | 152 | — | — |
| Liver | 360 | 662 | 848 | 1130 | 1200 |
| Kidney | 191.84 | 342 | 768 | — | — |
| Spleen | 108.15 | 127 | 156 | 224 | 260 |

Children who died of marasmus during the first two years of life showed marked reductions in cell number in all organs studied. As described in a preceding section, brain cell size was also reduced when the malnutrition extended into the second year. In contrast, cell size in the other organs was not significantly reduced even if the malnutrition persisted beyond the first year (Table 11).

## THEORETICAL CONSIDERATIONS

The data in the preceding sections have shown that the effects of malnutrition vary with the stage of cellular growth in any organ. During

**Table 11   DNA Content of Various Organs in Severe Marasmus (milligrams)**

| Months after Birth | 1.5 | 2.5 | 4 | 6 | 6.5 | 8 | 8.5 | 10 | 11 | 13 | 25 |
|---|---|---|---|---|---|---|---|---|---|---|---|
| Weight | 3450 | 3480 | 1900 | 2500 | 4000 | 4200 | 7100 | 4900 | 5300 | 9300 | 8500 |
| Brain | 630 | — | 306 | 329 | — | — | 767 | 744 | 602 | — | 847 |
| Heart | 42 | 44 | 16 | 27 | 30 | 52 | — | 39 | — | 53 | 114 |
| Liver | 244 | 292 | 198 | 180 | 224 | 364 | 397 | 393 | 384 | — | 885 |
| Kidney | 109 | 82 | 83 | — | — | 104 | 96 | 148 | — | 86 | 128 |
| Spleen | 56 | 30.5 | 68 | — | 174 | 57 | 29 | 151 | — | 260 | 198 |
| Adrenal | 5.26 | 5.86 | — | 1.1 | 4.2 | — | — | — | 1.67 | — | — |
| Thyroid | 5.93 | — | — | 1.5 | — | — | 4.3 | — | 3.5 | — | — |
| Right lung | 183 | — | — | — | 199 | 242 | — | — | — | — | 405 |

the stage of active DNA synthesis cell division is slowed. Later, protein/DNA ratios decrease. Both effects appear to be initiated by an interference with protein synthesis. Moreover, other stimuli influence cellular growth similarly. Hypothyroidism in the young animal produces a reduction in DNA content in those organs still undergoing active mitosis and reduces "cell size" in those in which cell division has already stopped (15). Other stimuli, such as clamping of the aorta (47) or uninephrectomy (64, 71), produce an increase in growth in the heart or contralateral kidney, respectively. In both situations the young animal responds with an increased amount of DNA synthesis, whereas the adult animal responds with an increase in RNA/DNA and protein/DNA ratios without cell division. Regardless of the final response of the tissue, either hyperplasia or hypertrophy, the early sequence of events is the same; for example, following uninephrectomy in adult rats, a series of changes in RNA metabolism occurs within one hour after the stimulus is applied. These changes result in active RNA synthesis, mainly ribosomal RNA and consequently an increase in RNA/DNA ratio (71). Either simultaneously or immediately thereafter the rate of protein synthesis also increases, and the result is an increase in the protein/DNA ratio (64, 71). In the young rat the sequence is identical, but after several hours of RNA and protein synthesis DNA synthesis begins and continues for several days (64).

The mechanisms by which the response to the same stimulus varies with age are unknown but would appear to be part of the more general phenomenon of cell differentiation, a major problem being investigated in the field of developmental biology. Ultimately these changes and those induced by malnutrition are reflecting changes in protein metabolism, and consequently the mechanisms that control the synthesis, regulation, and breakdown of protein must be considered responsible for many of the events that have been described during both normal and abnormal cellular growth.

Present knowledge suggests two possible mechanisms by which protein synthesis may be regulated: direct nuclear regulation of gene transcription and cytoplasmic regulation of translation from already formed templates.

The first possibility, based on the theory of Jacob and Monod, postulates the existence of an extensive number of specific cytoplasmic molecules (repressors) which pass from the cytoplasm into the nucleus and by attaching to specific loci inhibit the transcription of a particular gene or group of genes (62). The synthesis of DNA would then stop during development because the templates necessary for this process, among others perhaps the template for DNA polymerase, are no longer being transcribed. For certain organs (e.g., the brain or the kidney) this change is permanent and irreversible, whereas in other tissues (e.g., the liver) the possibility for reversal under specific conditions is maintained.

Strong evidence supports the possibility that a mechanism such as this is responsible for the "flexibility" that bacteria have in adapting to a new medium that lacks an essential nutrient or contains an inhibitory substance for some metabolic step. There is no clear evidence, however, for this mechanism in higher cells unless the RNA-DNA hybridization techniques are accepted as a source of information for mammalian cells. The data from these experiments are still questionable (12). Therefore, at least in the present "state of the art," there are few situations in which evidence for the suppression of a single gene or a group of genes in the mammal is convincing (11, 41, 69, 94). In all cases the final changes observed can be explained equally well by a second approach.

This second approach emphasizes the role of cytoplasmic mechanisms in the control of protein synthesis. Much of the evidence in favor of cytoplasmic regulation of the information elaborated in the nucleus comes from experiments done as early as 1926 in acetabularia, a giant unicellular alga. This cell grows and differentiates normally many weeks after the nucleus has been removed. Thus differentiation does not require a differential transcription of the genetic material. Moreover, in the already enucleated cell different levels of illumination can either maintain simple cell growth for a longer period or allow early differentiation (55). These observations suggest direct control of the cytoplasm over preexisting templates.

Continued differentiation in pancreatic cells of the mouse embryo and of hemoglobin-forming cells in the chick embryo after the administration of high doses of actinomycin D (82, 100) also favors the concept that certain decisive events of differentiation do not require concomitant gene activity. The ways in which these cytoplasmic regulatory mechanism operate, however, are a matter of pure speculation. Two possibilities are currently being considered; one involves configurational changes in the partly synthesized protein (91) and the other involves changes in transfer RNA (6).

We postulate that the effects of malnutrition are probably due to an interference with some of these mechanisms acting mainly at the cytoplasmic level. The cells of a "malnourished" tissue have less energy amino acids, and other nutrients available. This may alter ribosomal RNA metabolism or transfer RNA activity in some manner and, indirectly, affect protein synthesis.

The reduced RNA/DNA ratio observed in the malnourished adult animal is an index of the profound alterations that malnutrition induces in RNA metabolism. Few things are known about these changes, although it has been shown that the reduction in RNA/DNA ratio is due mainly to a reduction in ribosomal RNA content and that the mechanism of this reduction is an increased catabolic rate with apparently no changes in the rate of synthesis. There is also a more rapid turnover of tRNA and mRNA (78).

These changes in RNA metabolism are closely related to an increase in the activity of alkaline RNase, a cytoplasmic enzyme whose activity has been reported to be elevated during malnutrition (46). Other reports have shown that RNase activity varies during development in a number of organs (7, 17). Although the available data do not allow us to draw any general conclusions about the role of this enzyme, it is theoretically acceptable to conceive of RNase activity as a possible mechanism for the control of RNA metabolism, either by breaking down tRNA, rRNA, or mRNA in any combination or even by selectively breaking down different kinds of RNA.

The possibility that RNase could be participating in this mechanism prompted us to study this enzyme. To date, results indicate that alkaline RNase levels are increased in brain and liver of malnourished infant rats and that during normal development the activity per cell of the cytoplasmic fraction of this enzyme increases several fold. Activity per milligram of RNA, however, remains constant.

These developmental changes in RNase activity might interfere with translation of susceptible templates (e.g., DNA polymerase) without affecting others. Malnutrition further exaggerates these changes by elevating RNase activity. The increased activity of this enzyme, in turn, may selectively destroy certain templates or reduce the number of ribosomes available for translation. It is obvious that there are too few data for further speculation, and even the preceding explanation presents certain problems; for example, what controls RNase activity itself? Are the changes in development or with malnutrition a cause or a consequence of the events described? In addition, although alkaline RNase seems to be present in most higher cells, is the same pattern of activity present in all cells during development, malnutrition, or other adverse situations?

Investigations of the causes and mechanisms that induce changes in the activity of alkaline RNase and DNA polymerase are currently going on in our laboratory. It is hoped that they will help to bring about a better understanding of the mechanisms by which malnutrition interferes with the normal activities of the cell and by it a better understanding of the mechanism that regulates normal cell function.

## REFERENCES

1. C. W. M. Adams and A. N. Davison, *J. Neurochem.* **4:** 282 (1959).
2. G. A. O. Alleyne, *Clin. Sc. (London)* **34:** 199 (1968).
3. J. Altman, *J. Comp. Neurol.* **128:** 431 (1966).
4. J. Altman, in *Handbook of Neurochemistry,* A. Lajtha, Ed. New York: Plenum, 1969, p. 137.
5. J. Altman and G. Das, *J. Comp. Neurol.* **126:** 337 (1966).
6. B. N. Ames and P. E. Hartman, *Sympos. Quant. Biol.* (Cold Spring Harbor) **28:** 349 (1963).
7. J. D. S. Arora, and G. de Lamirande, *Canad. J. Biochem.* **45:** 1021 (1967).
8. K. B. Auguslinsson, in *The Enzymes: Chemistry and Mechanism of Action,* J. B. Sumner and Karl Myrback, Eds. New York: Academic, Vol. 1, 1950, p. 443.
9. R. K. Beach and J. L. Kostyo, *Endocrinology* **82:** 882 (1968).
10. P. Beaconsfield, J. Ginsburg, and M. Jeacock, *Develop. Med. Child Neurol.* **6:** 469 (1964).
11. L. Berlowitz, *Proc. Natl. Acad. Sci. (USA)* **53:** 68 (1965).
12. J. O. Bishop, *J. Biochem.* **116:** 223 (1970).
13. A. Boivin, R. Vendrely, and C. Vendrely, *Compt. Rend. Acad. Sci.* **226:** 1061 (1948).
14. G. Brante, *ACTA Physiol. Scand. (Suppl. 63)*, Stockholm, **18:** 1 (1949).
15. J. A. Brasel and M. Winick, *Growth* **34:** 197 (1970).
16. J. A. Brasel, R. A. Ehrenkranz, and M. Winick, *Develop. Biol.* **23:** 424, (1970).
17. S. Brody, *ACTA Biochim. Biophys.* **24:** 502 (1957).
18. R. P. Bunge, *Physiol. Rev.* **48:** 197 (1968).
19. H. P. Chase, J. Dorsey, and G. M. McKhann, *Pediat.* **40:** 551 (1967).
20. D. B. Cheek, in *Human Growth,* D. B. Cheek, Ed. Philadelphia: Lea & Febiger, 1968 p. 337.
21. D. B. Cheek, J. A. Brasel, D. Elliott, and R. Scott, *Bull. Johns Hopkins Hosp.* **119:** 46 (1969).
22. D. B. Cheek, J. A. Brasel, and J. E. Graystone, in *Human Growth,* D. B. Cheek, ed. Philadelphia: Lea & Febiger, 1968, p. 306.
23. D. B. Cheek, D. E. Hill, A. Cordano, and G. G. Graham, *Pediat. Res.* **4:** 135 (1970).
24. D. B. Cheek, A. B. Holt, D. E. Hill, and J. L. Talbert (in press).
25. D. B. Cheek, G. K. Powell, and R. E. Scott, *Bull. Johnn Hopkins Hosp.* **116:** 378 (1965).
26. E. L. Correy, *Amer. J. Physiol.* **112:** 263 (1935).
27. W. J. Culley, and R. Lineberger, *J. Nutr.* **96:** 375 (1968).
28. J. N. Cummings, H. Goodwin, E. M. Woodward, and G. Curzon, *J. Neurochem.* **2:** 289 (1958).
29. A. N. Davison and J. Dobbing, *Brit. Med. Bull.* **22:** 40 (1966).

30. A. N. Davison and J. Dobbing, in *Applied Neurochemistry*, A. N. Davison and J. Dobbing, Eds. Oxford: Blackwell Scientific Publications, 1968, p. 253.

31. J. W. T. Dickerson, J. Dobbing, and R. A. McCance, *Proc. Roy. Soc., London*, b166: 396, (1966–1967).

32. J. Dobbing and J. Sands, *Nature* 226: 639 (1970).

33. S. Duckett and A. G. Pearse, in *Proc. 5th Int. Congr. Neuropathology*, Pub. Excerpta Medica Foundation, Int. Congress Series, 100, 738 (1966).

34. S. Duckett and A. G. Pearse, *Canad. Rev. Biol.* 262: 173 (1967).

35. S. Duckett and A. G. Pearse, *J. Anat.* 102: 183 (1968).

36. S. Duckett and A. G. Pearse, *Anat. Rec.* 163: 59 (1969).

37. M. Enesco, *Anat. Rec.* 139: 225 (1961).

38. M. Enesco and C. P. Leblond, *J. Embryol. Exp. Morph.* 10: 530 (1962).

39. M. Enesco and D. Puddy, *Amer. J. Anat.* 114: 235 (1964).

40. C. J. Epstein, *Proc. Nat. Acad. Sci. (USA)* 57: 327 (1967).

41. H. J. Evans, C. E. Ford, M. F. Lyon, and J. Gray, *Nature* 206: 900 (1965).

42. I. Fish and M. Winick, *Pediat. Res.* 3: 407 (1969).

43. I. Fish and M. Winick, *Exp. Neurol.* 25: 534 (1969).

44. J. S. Garrow, K. Fletcher, and D. Halliday, *J. Clin. Invest.* 44: 417 (1965).

45. J. Ginsburg and M. Jeacock, *Biochem. Pharmacol.* 16: 497 (1967).

46. N. S. Girija, D. S. Pradham, and E. A. Sreenivasam, *Ind. J. Biochem.* 2: 85 (1965).

47. L. Gluck, N. J. Talner, H. Stern, T. H. Gardner, and M. V. Kulovich, *Science* 144: 1244 (1964).

48. E. E. Gordon, K. Kowalski, and M. Fritts, *Amer. J. Physiol.* 210: 1033 (1966).

49. G. G. Graham, A. Cordano, R. M. Blizzard, and D. B. Cheek *Pediat. Res.* 3: 579 (1969).

50. J. E. Graystone, in *Human Growth*, D. B. Cheek, Ed. Philadelphia: Lea & Febiger, 1968, p. 182.

51. J. E. Graystone and D. B. Cheek, *Pediat. Res.* 3: 66 (1969).

52. P. Gruenwald and H. N. Minn, *Amer. J. Obstet. Gynecol.* 82: 312 (1961).

53. D. C. Hagerman and C. A. Villee, *Physiol. Rev.* 40: 313 (1960).

54. D. Halliday, *Clin. Sci. (London)* 33: 365 (1967).

55. J. Hammerling, *Amer. Rev. Pl. Physiol.* 14: 65 (1963).

56. D. E. Hill, A. B. Holt, A. Parra, and D. B. Cheek, *Johns Hopkins Med. J.* 127: 146 (1970).

57. I. J. Holstein, W. A. Fish, and W. M. Stokes, *J. Lipid Res.* 7: 364 (1966).

58. L. E. Holt, R. McIntosh, and H. Barnett, in *Pediatrics*, 13th ed., L. E. Holt, R. McIntosh, and H. Barnett, Eds. New York: Appleton-Century-Crofts, 1962, p. 151.

59. E. Howard, D. M. Granoff, and P. Bujnovszky, *Brain Res.* 14: 697 (1969).

60. E. Howard and D. M. Granoff, *J. Nutr.* 95: 111 (1968).

61. C. M. Jackson and C. A. Steward, *J. Exper. Zool.* 30: 97 (1920).

62. F. Jacob and J. Monod, *J. Mol. Biol.* 3: 318 (1961).

63. W. P. Jollie, *Amer. J. Anat.* **114**: 161 (1964).

64. R. Karp, J. A. Brasel, and M. Winick, *Amer. J. Dis. Child.* **121**: 186 (1971).

65. D. Kritchevsky and W. L. Holmes, *Biochem. Biophys. Res. Commun.* **7**: 128 (1962).

66. L. W. Lapham, *Science* **159**: 310 (1968).

67. F. Le Baron, in *Handbook of Neurochemistry*, A. Lajtha, Ed. New York: Plenum, 1970, p. 561.

68. C. S. Lee and B. F. Chow, *J. Nutr.* **87**: 439 (1965).

69. U. C. Littan, U. G. Alfrey, J. H. Freuster, and A. E. Mirsky, *Proc. Natl. Acad. Sci. (USA)* **52**: 93 (1964).

70. J. F. Logan, W. A. Mannell, and R. Rossiter, *J. Biochem.* **51**: 482 (1952).

71. R. A. Malt, in *Compensatory Renal Hypertrophy*, W. W. Nowinsky, and R. J. Goss, Eds., New York: Academic, 1969, p. 131.

72. P. Mandel, H. Rein, S. Harth-Edel, and R. Mardell, in *Comparative Neurochemistry*, Derek Richter, Ed., London: Pergamon 1964, p. 153.

73. F. L. Margolis, *J. Neurochem.* **16**: 447 (1969).

74. S. A. Miller, in *Mammalian Protein Metabolism*, H. N. Munro and J. B. Allison, Eds., New York: Academic, Vol. 3, 1969, p. 189.

75. B. Nachmansohn, in *Modern Trends in Physiology and Biochemistry*, E. S. G. Barron, Ed., New York: Academic, 1952, p. 38.

76. B. S. Platt, *Proc. Roy. Soc.* (London) **156**: 337, (1962).

77. B. S. Platt, C. R. C. Heard, and R. J. C. Steward, in *Mammalian Protein Metabolism*, H. R. Munro, and J. B. Allison, Eds., New York: Academic, Vol. 2, 1964, Chapter 21.

78. C. Quirin-Stricker, and P. Mandel, *Bull. Soc. Chim. Biol.* **50**: 31 (1968).

79. G. H. Reem and N. Kretchmer, *Proc. Soc. Exptl. Biol. Med.* **96**: 458 (1957).

80. P. Rosso, J. Hormazbal, and M. Winick, *Amer. J. Clin. Nutr.* **23**: 1275 (1970).

81. G. Rouser and A. Yamamoto, in *Handbook of Neurochemistry*, A. Lajtha, Ed. New York: Plenum, 1969, p. 121.

82. W. J. Rutter, N. K. Wessells, and C. Grobstein, *J. Nat. Canc. Inst. Monogr. No. 13*, 51 (1964).

83. K. L. Standard, V. G. Willis, and J. C. Waterlow, *Amer. J. Clin. Nutr.* **7**: 271 (1959).

84. F. Sereni and O. Barnabei, personal communication, 1965.

85. C. A. Smith, *J. Pediat.* **30**: 229 (1947).

86. M. E. Smith, *Adv. Lipid Res.* **5**: 241 (1967).

87. W. Sperry, in *Neurochemistry*, K. A. C. Elliott, Irvine H. Page, and J. H. Quastel, Eds., Springfield, Illinois: 1962, p. 234.

88. L. Svennerholm, *J. Lipid Res.* **9**: 570 (1968).

89. A. H. Tingey, *J. Ment. Sc.* (London) **102**: 429 (1956).

90. F. E. Viteri and J. Alvarado, *Pediat.* **46**: 696 (1970).

91. H. J. Vogel, in *The Chemical Basis of Heredity*, W. D. McElroy and B. Glass, Eds., Baltimore: Johns Hopkins Press, 1957 p. 276.

92. J. C. Waterlow, *West Indian Med. J.* **5**: 167 (1956).

93. J. C. Waterlow and C. B. Mendes, *Nature* **180**: 1361 (1957).

94. J. M. Whitten, *Chromosoma* **26**: 215 (1969).

95. W. F. Widdas, *Brit. Med. Bull.* **17**: 107 (1961).

96. E. M. Widdowson, paper presented at the Symposium on Fetal Malnutrition, New York City, January 1970.

97. E. M. Widdowson and R. A. McCance, *Proc. Roy. Soc. (London)* **152**: 88 (1960).

98. H. Wiegardt, *J. Neurochem.* **14**: 671 (1967).

99. J. S. Wigglesworth, *J. Path. Bact.* **88**: 1 (1964).

100. F. H. Wilt, *J. Mol. Biol.* **12**: 331 (1965).

101. M. Winick, *J. Pediat.* **71**: 390 (1967).

102. M. Winick, in *Diagnosis and Treatment of Fetal Disorders,* K. Adamsons, Ed. New York: Springer 1968, p. 83.

103. M. Winick, *Pediat. Res.* **2**: 352 (1968).

104. M. Winick, *J. Nutr.* **94**: 121 (1968).

105. M. Winick, *Pediat. Clin. N. Amer.* **17**: 69 (1970).

106. M. Winick, *Fed. Proc.* **29**: 1510 (1970).

107. M. Winick, *Amer. J. Obstet. Gynecol.* **109**: 166 (1971).

108. M. Winick, A. Coscia, and A. Noble, *Pediat.* **39**: 248 (1967).

109. M. Winick, I. Fish, and P. Rosso, *J. Nutr.* **95**: 623 (1968).

110. M. Winick and P. Grant, *Endocrinology* **83**: 544 (1968).

111. M. Winick and A. Noble, *Develop. Biol.* **12**: 451 (1965).

112. M. Winick and A. J. Noble, *Nutr.* **89**: 300 (1966).

113. M. Winick and A. Noble, *Nature* **212**: 34 (1966).

114. M. Winick and A. Noble, *J. Nutr.* **91**: 179 (1967).

115. M. Winick and P. Rosso, *Pediat. Res.* **3**: 181 (1969).

116. M. Winick, P. Rosso, and J. Waterlow, *Exp. Neurol.* **26**: 393 (1970).

117. M. Winick and P. Rosso, paper presented to the Society for Clinical Nutrition (in press).

118. M. Winick, and E. Velasco, *Proc. 8th Int. Congr. Nutr.,* Prague, Czech., 1969 (in press).

119. S. Zamenof, E. Van Marthens, and F. L. Margolis, *Science* **160**: 3823 (1968).

120. F. S. Zeman and E. C. Stanbrough, *J. Nutr.* **99**: 274 (1969).

# 4

# Lipid Metabolism and Nutrition in the Prenatal and Postnatal Period

PETER HAHN*

Department of Obstetrics and Gynaecology and Department of Paediatrics, University of British Columbia, Vancouver General Hospital

All the information necessary for the synthesis of all the enzymes of the mature animal is stored in the conceived cell. This need not be true, but it is assumed to be so here. When and how certain enzymes and thus metabolic pathways first appear are determined by known and many unknown factors. Undoubtedly the quantity and quality of the nutrients supplied to the developing organism are important. It also appears that the quantity and quality of the food fed early in life decide the final makeup of the adult. The reasons are not clear. Certainly a good case could be made out for the following hypothesis: development is a one-way process. At the start many pathways are open to the developing organism which are determined by its genetic make-up. Once a certain pathway has been taken, however, all the other possible ones before that point are closed and development has to proceed along the chosen pathway. This can be easily demonstrated for morphological traits, say cleft palate, but it is much more difficult to show for less obvious characteristics. It is also true for mental functions (e.g., the learning of the first language and of all subsequent ones). This hypothesis can be put in a different way. The first adaptation to any environmental factor is the most important.

These highly hypothetical assumptions may help to explain some of the data recorded below.

This chapter was written with the financial support of M.R.C. Grant No. 68-3713.

* Medical Research Council (Canada) Associate.

Biochemical nutrition is really a tautological term, since all nutrition is essentially biochemical and all biochemistry in living matter is essentially dependent on nutrition. There are, however, smaller or larger barriers between externally supplied nutrients and biochemical processes in the various tissues. This may be illustrated by the fate of a triglyceride molecule after it has entered the gut. The mucosa of this organ is really the first tissue to encounter the molecule, and it may be expected that it will most directly relate biochemically to changes in diet, for example. The intestinal mucosa has to deal with the triglyceride supply in a biochemical fashion, partly hydrolyzing it with the aid of pancreatic lipase, absorbing it as glycerol and fatty acids and monoglycerides into the villi, reesterifying it, and channeling the short-chain fatty acids and glycerol into the liver and the long-chain fatty acids mostly as reconstituted triglycerides into the lymph. It follows that the second organ most directly in contact with external nutrients is the liver and, in the case of long-chain fatty acids, other peripheral organs with adipose tissue and liver being the most prominent (although the heart and lungs are the first to encounter these compounds). Hence it is not surprising that biochemical changes due to changes in diet composition are most pronounced in liver and adipose tissue and that they are equally striking in the small intestine, even though this organ has received much less attention (1). Other organs are less susceptible to dietary influences, since their supply of nutrients is relatively buffered, so to speak, by the liver and adipose tissue.

The above is valid for adult animals. In the fetus a different situation prevails. All food is supplied via the placenta, which plays an active part in the regulation of transfer of nutrients, whereas the liver and particularly the gut of the fetus are apparently of little importance for nutrient absorption at that time.

## THE FETUS

### Fatty Acid Oxidation

It has been stated repeatedly that fetal nutrition via the placenta in all mammals studied so far can be called a "high carbohydrate" diet (2, 3). The main nutrient passed from mother to fetus is glucose, but it is probable that products of glycolysis are also utilized. Lipids are oxidized only to a small extent by fetal organs. Surprisingly enough, this assumption has been verified to a limited extent only and, in fact, excepting the work of Hahn and Vavrouskova (4) in man and of Drahota et al. (5) in the rat, we are not aware of any work in this field.

Hahn and Vavrouskova showed that the liver of human fetuses aged about 12 weeks after conception is capable of producing ketone bodies from oleic acid in vitro but that this capacity is limited and that the concentration of oleic acid in the medium to produce such an effect is fairly high. It was also found that isolated mitochondria from fetal human liver do not produce any ketone bodies at all from oleic acid. Perhaps the production of these substances is extramitochondrial, a possibility suggested by Sauer for guinea pig liver (6). Ketone body production in the rat by fetal liver could not be demonstrated and was initiated only after birth (5). Recently we have examined it in more detail in the human fetus. In all the organs studied the rate of oxidation of palmitic acid by homogenates are very low and only slightly affected by the addition of carnitine and coenzyme A (Hahn, unpublished). Thus it seems that the fetus is not equipped to any extent for the oxidation of fatty acids and for the formation of ATP by fatty acid breakdown. Teleologically speaking, this is understandable, since the oxygen requirement for fatty acid oxidation is much greater than that for glucose utilization.

Why is fatty acid oxidation so low in the fetus? Here we can only speculate, since there is only one paper dealing with this problem. The heart of the newborn rat lacks carnitine and acylcarnitine transferase and it takes about 10 days of postnatal development for the mechanisms of fatty acid oxidation to develop (7) (Fig. 1). It is tempting to ascribe the postnatal development to induction by the high level of fatty acids in the blood as suggested by the investigators, but there is no direct proof.

Another reason for the low rate of fatty acid oxidation in the fetus might be sought in mitochondrial development itself, since so far this process is thought to occur only in these cell particles. Again data are scanty indeed and, as far as fatty acid oxidation goes, nonexistent. Undoubtedly mitochondria change morphologically and biochemically during fetal development (8). It has been shown, for instance, that the localization of phosphoenopyruvate carboxykinase is intramitochondrial in the fetus and mainly extramitochondrial after birth (9).

It must also be stressed that, particularly in the human fetus but also in other species, our knowledge is usually limited to a certain period of fetal development and that changes during fetal development are known only to a limited extent. Thus the low rate of fatty acid oxidation in human fetuses was found in specimens aged 10 to 20 weeks and this need not be true for earlier or later periods of development.

Another reason for the low rate of fatty acid oxidation in the fetus might be sought in the diet it consumes. It is well established that

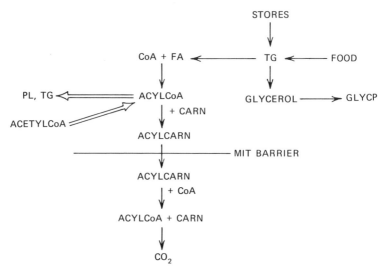

**Fig. 1.** A supply of fatty acids (*FA*) for oxidation: *mit* = mitochondrial, *CoA* = coenbyme *A*, *carn* = carnitine, *PL* = phospholipid, *TG* = triglycerides, *Glyc P* = glycerophosphate. Pathways shown by boldface arrows develop after birth. Pathways shown by light arrows are inhibited after birth, at least in the liver.

a high carbohydrate diet supports fatty acid synthesis rather than fatty acid oxidation and our biochemical knowledge of the fetus is in good agreement with this fact. In all species examined so far glycolysis has been found to be well in evidence. The pentose shunt is operative (10) and the rate of gluconeogenesis (11, 12) is low or absent (see below). This is particularly true of the liver (the organ most frequently studied) (Fig. 2).

All the evidence in adult animals supports the contention that such a metabolic situation is conducive to fatty acid synthesis and indicates that fatty acid oxidation is low or not occurring at all.

## Fatty Acid Synthesis

In the fetus, as might be expected, fatty acid synthesis is well in evidence (13, 14 for rats, 15 for man, 16, 17 for rabbits). Again we must caution the reader that "fetus" is rather a vague term, since we do not know how valid our data are for the whole fetal period. In the rat, for instance, the rate of fatty acid synthesis is higher just before birth than two to four days earlier (13).

As already mentioned, the pentose shunt is active in the fetus (10) and, in fact, is more active than later in life (18). Hence NADPH requirements for fatty acid synthesis seem to be met. Direct evidence of fatty acid synthesis has been submitted repeatedly in both man and rat from glucose, pyruvate, acetate, and citrate (14).

It seems, however, that fatty acid synthesis develops in the rat fetus (14) and that in the very young human fetus it is lower than in the older ones (15). A more detailed examination of the mechanisms involved shows that simple explanations of development are not valid (Fig. 2).

If we accept that one of the mechanisms of fatty acid synthesis from glucose involves the citrate cleavage pathway, i.e., transport of acetyl-CoA out of the mitochondria in the form of citrate, which is then broken down to oxalo-acetate and acetyl-CoA, and we further accept that malic

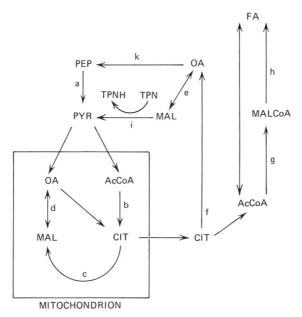

Fig. 2. A diagram to show metabolic pathways for pyruvate oxidation and fatty acid synthesis: *PEP* = phosphoenolpyruvate, *PYR* = pyruvate, *OA* = oxaloacetic acid, *MAL* = malate, *cit* = citrate, *AcCoA* = acetylCoA, *MALCoA* = malonylCoA, *FA* = fatty acid. The small letters indicate enzymes: (a) pyruvate kinase, (b) citrate synthase, (c) Krebs cycle sequence, (d) malic dehydrogenase, (e) malic dehydrogenase (cytoplasmic), (f) citrate lyase, (g) acetylCoA carboxylase, (h) fatty acid synthetase, (i) malic enzyme, (j) phosphoenol pyruvate carboxykinase. Synthesis of oxaloacetate from pyruvate is ensured by pyruvate carboxylase. In most mammalian fetuses enzymes (k) and (i) show little activity. After birth (k) rapidly increases and the activities of (a), (f), (g), and (h) are decreased. During weaning they and (i) increase again.

enzyme is important to fatty acid synthesis by supplying NADPH and pyruvate, we can discuss the known data from this aspect.

In fetal rat liver the activity of citrate cleavage enzyme is high, about as high as in the adult (13, 19). Again, the age of the fetus may be important. The youngest fetuses examined were 18 days old. In the human fetal liver no citrate cleavage enzyme could be demonstrated in fetuses younger than 20 weeks (Hahn, unpublished), which is in good agreement with the fact that fatty acid synthesis from labeled citrate can first be demonstrated somewhat later (15). In contrast to the liver fatty acid synthesis in fetal human brain never seems to be via the citrate cleavage pathway (15). Only labeled acetate is utilized. Malic enzyme has low activity in fetal liver, both in rats and humans, and this condition can be related to the fact that gluconeogenesis and cytoplasmic phosphoenolpyruvate carboxykinase are not demonstrable and thus oxalo-acetate is available to malic enzyme only (13) (see Fig. 2). Hence the low activity of malic enzyme present in fetal liver appears to be sufficient to support the citrate pathway of fatty acid synthesis. From the nutritional point of view the ruminant fetus is of special interest. Its supply of glucose from the mother is evidently insufficient to cover its energy requirements, and as a result gluconeogenesis in its liver does occur (13) (in ox fetuses, for instance, malic enzyme activity is high, higher than in adults, and liver citrate lyase activity is abundant, but negligible in adults). It would be interesting to correlate these findings in more detail with the supply of nutrients to the fetal ox. Among other things, it is surprising to find gluconeogenesis and fatty acid synthesis side by side.

Even though we know more about fatty acid synthesis than about fatty acid oxidation in the fetus, we are still a long way from understanding all the mechanisms involved. The problem of transfer of fatty acids from mother to fetus is still open to many speculations and the calculations put foward are tentative indeed. Here species differences will also play an important role.

### Fatty Acid Supply from the Mother

If we assume that fatty acid oxidation is negligible, we can make an attempt to calculate the rate of fatty acid supply obtained from the mother by the fetus itself. Let us assume that the rat fetus, aged 16 days, doubles its weight in 28 hours (20). Thus its weight would increase by 460 mg or about 16 mg/hr. Since the lipid content of the rat fetus is about 1% (20), this would mean an increase of 0.16 mg of fat during that period. Most of the lipid is phospholipid (21), and the amount of fatty acid accumulated would thus be about 0.1 mg, which is about

0.4 $\mu$mole. The liver of a 16-day-old fetus weighs about 80 mg and the rate of fatty acid synthesis calculated from the data of Hanson and Ballard (13) would be 0.36 $\mu$mole/liver-hour. This leaves 0.04 $\mu$mole unaccounted for, but since the rest of the fetus also synthetises FA it would seem that no transport of fatty acids is required. A similar calculation by Villee (22) also came to the same conclusions.

On the other hand, it has been shown repeatedly that fatty acids are transported from mother to the fetus in rats (23), rabbits (24), guinea pigs (25), sheep (26), man (24, 27), and monkeys (28). In fact, one calculation claims that this supply is sufficient to account for all the fatty acids in the fetus (26) (for a review see 29). It has also been shown that the isolated human term placenta can transfer fatty acids from the maternal to the fetal circulation and, even though to a lesser extent, also in the opposite direction (27). Nevertheless, quantitative data are hard to come by and the rate of transfer of fatty acids differs between species, apparently being low in rats and sheep and high in guinea pigs and monkeys (Tables 1 and 2), where it increases

#### Table 1   Effect of Gestational Age on Sixty-Minute Transfer of Linoleic $^{14}$C-1 Acid from Maternal Blood to Fetus in the Monkey

|                  | Dpm/g Fetal Tissue |
|------------------|--------------------|
| Gestational Age  | Injected Dose      |
| 37               | 0.010              |
| 54               | 0.038              |
| 60               | 0.14               |
| 150+             | 0.70               |

Adapted from Portman et al. (28)

#### Table 2   Effect of Fasting on Fatty Acid Content of Maternal and Fetal Plasma in the Guinea Pig (mg/l)[a]

|          | Fed | 36-Hour Fast |
|----------|-----|--------------|
| Maternal | 140 | 980          |
| Fetal    | 210 | 960          |

[a] Adapted from Hershfield and Nemeth (25).

with increasing fetal age. It is tacitly assumed that essential fatty acids must reach the fetus from the mother and that the fetus cannot synthetize them. This is borne out by older experiments, even though only to some degree (27). On the other hand, it has been concluded that, except perhaps for the liver, the rat fetus synthetizes all its own fat (14).

If we apply rather vague calculations to the near-term human fetus and assume that the rate of umbilical plasma flow is 180 ml/min (31) and that the maternal plasma contains 0.6 meq of fatty acids per liter (32), potentially the fetus could extract $180 \times 0.06 \times 60 \times 24$ meq fatty acids-155 meq/day, which is equivalent to 38.9 g of fatty acid per day. Since the human fetus lays down 14 g of fat per day during the last month of gestation (20) and about 10 of the 14 g are fatty acids, the rate of fatty acid extraction from the mother by the fetus would have to be about 30% or 7 mg/min or about 25 $\mu$eq/min. Now let us consider that the total plasma volume of a 3-kg fetus is 150 ml. The level of fatty acid in fetal blood is only about 0.3 meq/l, and thus the total amount of fatty acids in the fetal plasma is about 45 $\mu$eq. In order for all the fatty acids to be transported from mother to fetus, the difference in the concentration of fatty acids in the umbilical vein and the umbilical artery would have to be 0.13 meq/l. If we take a more realistic figure of fat accumulation, as suggested by Sabata et al. (31), i.e., 2.4 g of fat accumulated per day during the last seven weeks of pregnancy, the arterial venous difference in the fetus would have to be only 0.02 meq/l. Such a difference is not easy to demonstrate by present-day methods of fatty acid determination. This, of course, would be the maximum amount of fatty acids retained and, since there is no doubt that fatty acid synthesis occurs in the fetus, it still remains a moot point whether, and how much, fatty acid is actually transferred from mother to fetus. Whatever the final answer it must be borne in mind that in contrast to glucose the fatty acid level in the mother's blood is usually not reflected in that of the fetus (13). It is possible to raise the fatty acid level in the rat maternal plasma by a factor of 2 to 4 (e.g., diabetes), yet there is no increase in the level of fatty acids in fetal blood (14). In the rat starvation plus diabetes in the mother suppresses FA synthesis in the late fetus but not in its brain (14). Nevertheless, there are some reports that even in man the rate of FA transport from mother to fetus can be raised by raising the FA level in the maternal blood (31). On the whole this is a different situation than holds for glucose transfer, in which, as the level of glucose increases in the mother, it also increases in the fetus. In the same way a rise in the level of ketone bodies in the mother's blood is reflected

in a similar rise in the human fetus (33) and the rat (34) but not
the sheep (35). Hence on balance it would seem that the transfer of
fatty acids from mother to fetus is not considerable and that probably
most of the fatty acids are produced by the fetus itself. Nevertheless,
we are quite prepared, if further evidence is forthcoming, to change
our opinion on this point.

## Cholesterol

As in the case of triglycerides and phospholipids, cholesterol esters do
not cross the placenta from the mother to the fetus (29, 36). It appears,
however, that free cholesterol is transported to some extent (38), but
much work remains to be done in this respect. Among other things,
it would be important to know the mechanisms that channel acetylCoA
into fatty acid or cholesterol synthesis. We are not aware of any study
that examines developmental changes in beta-hydroxy, beta-methyl-
butyryl CoA synthetase, or reductase nor of the effect of dietary changes
in the development of these enzymes. Until more is known speculations
will remain sterile. At the moment it appears that, as in the case of
phospholipids, the placenta plays an important role in the esterification
of cholesterol (36).

## Triglycerides

It is interesting to note that the triglyceride content of the newborn
of different species varies considerably. In rats, hamsters, and kittens
there is little fat in the body at birth, whereas in others (e.g., man
or guinea pigs) the fat content is abundant. Yet the fetuses of all mammals go through a period in which they have hardly any triglyceride
in their bodies and the little that is found is in liver and adrenals but
apparently nowhere else (Novak and Jirasek, personal communication).
The deposition of triglycerides in adipose tissue and perhaps elsewhere
occurs only toward the end of pregnancy in man and other mammals
born with a considerable amount of triglyceride in their bodies. We
do not know whether these triglycerides are formed from fatty acids,
transported from the mother or from fatty acids synthetised in the fetus.
What is fairly well established is that triglycerides do not cross the
placental barrier in any species studied so far (29).

The triglyceride level of the blood of the fetus is generally low. It
does not reflect the triglyceride level in maternal blood and is not
affected by starvation, overfeeding, or hormonal influences in the mother
(39 for review). In the fetal rabbit and guinea pig triglyceride blood

levels and triglyceride liver content are much higher than in human, rat, and sheep fetuses and, in fact, are higher than the levels found in their mothers (39). Some procedures will raise the triglyceride content of the liver of rat fetuses, but the fat content of the carcass is hardly affected (14, 40). There are only speculations concerning the origin of these additional triglycerides. Some authors assume increased transplacental supply of fatty acids (41); others suggest fat mobilization by the fetus itself (42). In late human fetuses about which little is known the latter process could be operative, since there is sufficient fatty acid present in adipose tissue and lipolysis can evidently be induced by hypoxia and other mechanisms (42). It is difficult, however, to consider such a mechanism in rats, since they have no fat in their white adipose tissue prenatally and the fat content of their brown adipose tissue is also small. In addition, there is another difficulty in explaining the increased fat content in fetal liver after various stresses. Whatever the origin of the fatty acids used for the synthesis of liver triglycerides, glycerol is also required and that can probably come only from glucose. Hence it must be postulated that under such conditions not only are fatty acids supplied to the liver but also the liver has available mechanisms and substrate for the synthesis of triglycerides. In rat fetuses, however, the activities of glycerol kinase and glycerophosphate dehydrogenase are very low (43, 10), and utilization of glycerol by the human newborn is lower than by older infants (Table 3), so that it

**Table 3   Glycerol Utilization by Human Infants**[a]

|  | Newborn | Three to Five Weeks Old |
| --- | --- | --- |
| Half-life of glycerol in blood | 39.9 min | 12.0 min |
| Percent rise in blood glucose, 30 min after glycerol infusion | +11.5% | +12.6% |

[a] Adapted from Wolf et al. (11).

seems unlikely that they could ensure a sufficient supply of $\alpha$-glycerophosphate for phospholipids and triglyceride synthesis. The only organ found so far with very high glycerophosphate dehydrogenase activity in man is the fetal intestinal mucosa (44), and it is possible that phospholipids and triglycerides are synthetized here in the fetus. This suggestion is supported by the fact that the human fetal colon contains many lipid droplets (45) and that triglyceride synthesis via both the mono-glyceride and the $\alpha$-glycerophosphate pathways is higher in the gut of fetal lambs than that of newborn or adults (46) (Table 4).

Table 4    Rate of Triglyceride Synthesis in Sheep Intestine[a]

| | Monoglyceride Pathway | $\alpha$-Glycero-Phosphate Pathway |
|---|---|---|
| | ($\mu$moles/100 mg) | |
| Fetal | 13 | 68 |
| Newborn | 13 | 54 |
| Adult | 8 | 35 |

[a] Adapted from Ref. 80.

## Phospholipids

There is general agreement that phospholipids do not cross the placenta (39). Injection of doubly labeled phospholipids into the mother results in the transfer of individual components to the fetus, and these are then found in fetal phospholipids whose fatty acid composition differs considerably from that of the compounds originally injected. It has been suggested that the phospholipids from the maternal circulation are broken down in the placenta and that new ones are formed there which are then handed over to the fetus by the placenta (47). As mentioned above, it is also possible that some of the fetal phospholipids are synthetized in the small intestine and phospholipid synthesis certainly occurs in fetal liver and lung. In fact, the rate of synthesis of choline glycero-phosphatides in fetal rat liver just before delivery is very high (48), whereas most other parameters of phospholipid synthesis reach a peak in the liver about 10 days after birth (48, 49). There are also consider-able differences in the rate of phospholipid synthesis between fetal and newborn lung which have been studied in both rat and lamb (50, 51). This is a special subject as far as lungs are concerned and the interested reader is referred to Ref. 52.

## AFTER BIRTH

### Perinatal Period

A 3-kg baby has a liver weighing 120 g and containing approximately 10 g of glycogen, which is equivalent to 40 large calories. If all this glycogen were to be used up, it would last (assuming a caloric requirement of 80 calories/day-kg in the newborn infant) one-sixth of a day, or four hours. Let us add 1 g/100 g of glycogen in muscle. Assume that the infant has 600 g of muscle (i.e., 6 g of glycogen, or 24 calories). This would give another two hours for the newborn infant. This is true only if all the glycogen is used up, which it is not (53). A good guess would be that the baby could live on its own glycogen stores for three to four hours after birth. For that period there would be no need to mobilize endogenous fat.

There are other considerations, however. *Glucose-6-phosphatase*, the enzyme responsible for releasing glucose from glucose-6-phosphate, becomes active only after birth (54) in most species; hence a certain period of time would be expected to elapse before glycogen is converted to glucose in the liver. Liver and brain phosphorylase activity is also said to be low in the rat fetus (55, 56), and so this would be another handicap to glycogen utilization in the newborn. In addition, the level of blood glucose is lower than in older infants and adults, not only in the fetus but also in the newborn, which indicates that the rate of glucose release from the liver is certainly low, since glucose utilization at that time of life is decreased (2, 53, 57). (The changes occurring during development are listed in Table 5).

It has been known for a decade that after delivery the blood level of free fatty acids increases rapidly in the newborn (26, 58, 59, Table 6), and it has been assumed that this was due to (a) sympathetic stimulation of lipolysis in adipose tissue (26) and (b) to the period of starvation that occurs after birth (58). Now it has been suggested that most of this postnatal rise is due to exposure to low environmental temperatures (59, 60, 61, 62, 63) (Table 7).

It is probable that all three factors play a role:

1. The rapid postnatal rise in blood level of free fatty acids can be inhibited by sympatholytic agents (64).

2. The level of free fatty acids reaches a peak within 6 to 24 hours after birth (58), indicating that sympathetic stimulation of lipolysis is probably not the only fact and that this prolonged elevation of the free fatty acid level may be ascribed to starvation and lack of glucose.

3. The level of free fatty acids, but more particularly the level of glycerol, rises considerably in cold-exposed newborns (63), suggesting that part of the adipose tissue at least (see below) is indirectly sensitive to cold in so far as noradrenaline release at sympathetic nerve endings in response to cold is concerned. This leads to lipolysis and release of glycerol and to some extent free fatty acids.

**Table 5  Metabolic Change in the Perinatal Period**

| Fetus | Premature Newborn | Postmature Fetus | Suckling | Weaned | Function | Species | Organ | Reference |
|---|---|---|---|---|---|---|---|---|
| 0 | ↑ | | ← | → ↑ | Ketone production | Rat | Liver | 5 |
| ↑ | ↓ | ↑ | → | ↑ | FA synthesis | Man, rat, rabbit | Liver, adipose tissue | 9, 12, 13, 15, 16, 83 |
| ← | | | → | ← | Acetyl CoA carboxylase | Rat | Liver, adipose tissue | 83 |
| ← | | | → | ← | Citrate cleavage | Rat | Liver, adipose tissue | 19 |
| ← | | | → | ← | Acetyl CoA synthesis | Rat | Liver, adipose tissue | 19 |
| ← | | | ← | → | FA synthesis | Rat | Brain | 124 |
| ← | | | → | → | Glycolysis | Rat | Liver, muscle | |
| 0 | ↑ | | ← | ↑ | Gluconeogenesis | Rat | Liver | 12, 13 |
| 0 | | 0 | ← | → | Carnitine–acetyl CoA transfer | Rat | Heart | 7 |
| → | | | → | → | FFA glycerol content | Rat, man | Blood | 2 |
| → | | | ← | → | TG, cholesterol, ketones | Rat, man | Blood | 2 |
| → | | | → | ← | Hormone sensitive lipase | Rat | Adipose tissue | 19 |
| → | | | ← | → | Lipoprotein lipase | Rat | Adipose tissue | 19 |
| → | | | → | ↓ ← | Lipase | Rat | Liver, brain, heart, pancreas, gut | 2, 115 |
| | | | ← | → | AMP phosphodiesterase[a] | Rat | Adipose tissue[a] | 2 |
| → ← | | | ← | → | Fat supply | Most mammals | | 2 |
| | | | → | ← | Glucose supply | Most mammals | | 2 |
| → | | | ← | → | Glycerokinase | Rat | Adipose tissue | 43 |
| → | | | ← | ← | Glycerokinase | Rat | Liver | 11 |
| | | | ← | ↑ | GPDH | Rat | Liver | 10 |

[a] unpublished results

111

Table 6 **Plasma Content of Fatty Acids and Lipoprotein Lipase of Mother, Fetus, and Newborn of Various Species**

| | Mother | Fetus (u.a.) | Fetus (u.v.) | Newborn | One Month | Species | Reference |
|---|---|---|---|---|---|---|---|
| FA meq/l | 1.84 | 0.65 | 0.56 | | | Man | 95 |
| | 1.25 | 0.27 | 0.29 | | | Man | 31 |
| | | | 0.28 | 0.95 | | Man | 2 |
| | 0.5 | 0.3 | 0.3 | 0.9 (fasted)<br>0.5 (glucose) | 0.95 | Man | 65 |
| | 0.59 | 0.39 | 0.39 | 0.43 (section)<br>0.90 (normal) | | Rabbit | 60 |
| | 0.8 | 0.5 | 0.5 | 1.0 | 1.6 (10 days) | Rat | 2 |
| | 1.0 | 0.2 | 0.2 | 0.6 (warm)<br>1.2 (cold) | | Lamb | 35 |
| Lipoprotein lipase units/l | 3.50 | 3.30 | | 550 (fasted)<br>260 (glucose) | | Man | 65 |

Table 7 Plasma Free Fatty Acid Levels in Newborn Rabbits Kept at 36–37°C[a]

| | Serum FFA (mg l) |
|---|---|
| Maternal | 0.59 |
| Fetal at term | 0.39 |
| Newborn, 24 hours | |
| Caesarean section (not fed) | 0.43 |
| Newborn, 24–30 hours | |
| Natural delivery (fed) | 0.90 |
| Ten-day-old rats (fed) | 1.6[b] |
| (starved) | 0.8[b] |

[a] Adapted from Hardman and Hull (59)
[b] Hahn and Koldovsky (2)

4. The high level of free fatty acids can be lowered by glucose infusions (2) and raised by fasting, again supporting the theory that lack
of glucose is responsible for free fatty acid release. In addition, lipoprotein lipase activity in the blood of newborns is also decreased by
glucose feeding (65).

These, to some extent contradictory, conclusions can be viewed with
fewer misgivings if we stipulate the presence of two types of adipose
tissue in the newborn.

## Adipose Tissue

One type, the normal white adipose tissue, is responsible for storage
and release of lipids. These processes are dependent on the prevailing
nutritional situation. The other, the brown adipose tissue, is related to
heat production and thus to maintenance of a stable body temperature.
After delivery it seems likely that the early increase in the level of
free fatty acids and glycerol is due to stimulation of lipolysis in brown
adipose tissue induced by the cooling usually accompanying exit from
the maternal environment. The later maintained elevation of the level
of free fatty acids in the blood, on the other hand, is probably a nutritional phenomenon explicable by a relative lack of glucose and insulin
resulting in lipolysis in white adipose tissue (Fig. 3). Changes occurring
in white adipose tissue of newborn infants all agree with this supposition.
Soon after birth the rate of incorporation of fatty acids into triglycerides

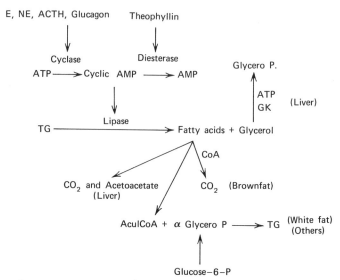

Fig. 3. A scheme of mechanisms of lipolysis. The lipase that breaks down triglycerides is activated by cyclic AMP, and the formation of cyclic AMP is induced by an adenyl-cyclase activated by epinephrine, norepinephrine, ACTH glucagon, and other agents. The fatty acids can be oxidized to $CO_2$, used to reform triglycerides, or oxidized to acetoacetate. The glycerol released on lipolysis has to be reactivated to glycerol phosphate before it can be used for triglyceride synthesis. Glycerol phosphate is formed either from glycerol by glycerokinase or from dihydroxyacetone phosphate by glycerophosphate dehydrogenase. In suckling rats the hormone-sensitive lipase of brown and white adipose tissue shows low activity (19) and the sensitivity of the lipase toward ACTH and glucagon is decreased (116).

is depressed (66), the content of fatty acids and glycerol is increased (67), and the oxygen consumption is higher and raised more by norepinephrine than later in life. Palmitate oxidation is also greater (68).

Nevertheless, in newborn babies we assume that brown adipose tissue functions only in the way we known it to function in other newborn mammals. Thus we can extrapolate only from our knowledge in the laboratory, and we must still make assumptions because we do not know enough about the human. No data on the biochemical development of human brown adipose tissue are available. It disappears gradually in man and other mammals as the animal gets older and is particularly prominent in hibernators or in cold-exposed rats (69). Its presence in newborn babies has been demonstrated both morphologically (70, 71) and by means of skin-temperature measurements between the shoulder blades (71). The most striking feature of brown adipose tissue in newborn rats, rabbits, guinea pigs, and other mammals is the presence of a large number of mitochondria which contain highly packed cristae. Discussion is still going on whether these mitochondria are coupled under normal conditions, and it is not the task of this review to enter into details. The interested reader is referred to Smith and Horwitz (69).

Our present state of knowledge indicates that brown adipose tissue produces heat that warms up the blood passing through it on its way to vital centers of the body (brain and heart). How this heat is produced is being studied intensively in several laboratories. It is fairly well established that mitochondria from brown adipose tissue preferentially oxidizes fatty acids. These fatty acids themselves probably in some way uncouple oxidative phosphorylation, particularly in newborn animals (73, 74), and thus the energy produced during fatty acid oxidation is dissipated as heat and is not used to any large extend for ATP formation. Since brown adipose tissue is typical for newborn mammals and hibernants, it is pertinent to discuss it in more detail here.

Just as in white adipose tissue, lipolysis is induced in brown adipose tissue by sympathetic stimulation, and it is not quite clear what stimuli induce lipolysis in brown and in white adipose tissue, since the former reacts to cold, whereas the latter reacts to lack of calories, at least in rabbits (74). In any case the fate of the hydrolyzed triglycerides (i.e., glycerol and fatty acids) is not the same in brown as in white adipose tissue (Fig. 3). White adipose tissue releases most of the fatty acids and glycerol produced and retains only sufficient fatty acids to reesterify them, whereas in brown adipose tissue, although reesterification of fatty acids also takes place, their main fate is to be oxidized by the mitochondria and not to be released into the circulation. That is the reason why on cold exposure of newborn infants the blood contains a large amount of glycerol and much less fatty acid (63), particularly in dysmature newborns.

Our knowledge of biochemical development in both brown and white adipose tissue is meagre (Tables 8 and 9), particularly in the human being. It is essentially true that we know next to nothing about the effect of diet on white and brown adipose tissue in the early postnatal period in both man and mammals. In fact, data are so scarce that a concentrated effort in this area should supply us with much new and valuable information. At the moment there is considerably indirect evidence that the change in diet induced by delivery and weaning does affect biochemical processes in both brown and white adipose tissue, just as nutritional changes in adult animals produce changes in liver and white adipose tissue (no one has looked at the effect of diet in adult animals on brown adipose tissue probably because brown adipose tissue is rare and often nonexistent in such animals).

**Table 8  Developmental Changes in Brown Adipose Tissue**

| | Fetus | Newborn | 5 Days | 17 Days | 3 to 4 Weeks | Species | Reference | Units |
|---|---|---|---|---|---|---|---|---|
| P/O pyr → mal | 0.5 | 0.47 | | | 2.6 | Guinea pig | 73 | $O_2$/min/mg prot |
| P/O succin | 1.0 | 0.08 | | | 0.05 | Guinea pig | 73 | |
| Mito.$O_2$ cons | | 154 | 280 | | 205 | Rat | 127 | |
| Percent body weight | | 0.7 | 0.6 | 0.3 | 0.2 | Rat | 125 | |
| | | 1.4 | 0.5 | 0.5 | 0.5 | Mouse | 125 | |
| | | 0.6 | 0.4 | 0.25 | 0.2 | Lemming | 125 | |
| | | 0.1 | 0.15 | 0.4 | 0.6 | Hamster | 125 | |
| | 5.5 | 3.0 | | | | Rabbit | 125 | |
| | 3.0 | 2.7 | | | | Guinea pig | 125 | |
| Percent protein | | 10.5 | 11.2 | 13.0 | 17.3 | Rat | 119 | |
| Percent fat | | 16.0 | | 40 | 58 | Rat | 119 | |
| SDH | | 0.142 | 0.195 | 0.237 | 0.186 | Rat | 120, 121 | $\mu$mol min-mg |
| GPDH (mito) | | 0.092 | 0.167 | 0.203 | 0.134 | Rat | 120, 121 | |
| COX | | 0.424 | 0.533 | 0.659 | 0.545 | Rat | 120, 121 | Protein |
| Malic enzyme | | 0.02 | 0.024 | 0.02 | 0.02 | Rat | 121 | Protein |
| GPDH (cytopl) | | 3.5 | 2.8 | 2.2 | 1.9 | Rat | 122 | $\mu$mole/min-mg |
| GAPDH | | 2.2 | 1.8 | 1.7 | 1.3 | Rat | 122 | Protein |
| Citrate cleavage | 2.0 | 2.0 | 0.4 | 0.8 | 3.5 | Rat | 122 | Protein |
| Acetyl CoA synth | | 0.6 | 0.3 | 0.3 | 0.9 | Rat | 19 | $\mu$mole/40 min-mg prot |
| Acetyl CoA carbox | 0.02 | | 0.01 | 0.01 | 0.22 | Rat | 19 | $\mu$mole/40 min-mg prot |
| Hormone sensitive lipase | | | | | | Rat | 124 | $\mu$mole/30 min-mg prot |
| Acetate → fatty acid | | 2.3 | 3.0 | | 8.0 | Rat | 19 | $\mu$eqFA/20 ft/mg prot |
| Glycerol → TG | | | 700 | | 1800 | Rat | 124 | $\mu$mole/mg prot/min |
| | | | 4000 | | 1900 | Rat | 11 | cpm/mg fat/120 min. |

Abbreviations: pyr = pyruvate, mal = malate, succin = succinate, mito = mitochondrial, cons = consumption, SDH = succinic dehydrogenase, GPDH = glycerophosphate dehydrogenase, COX = cytochromeoxidase, cytopl = cytoplasmic, GAPDH = glyceraldehydedehydrogenase, synth = synthetase, carbox = carboxylase, TG = triglyceride, prot = protein.

**Table 9    Composition of White Adipose Tissue of Man**

| | Lip- ids | Water (%) | Nitro- gen (%) | DNA (mg/g) | Cells/g | FA Percent of Total FA | | |
|---|---|---|---|---|---|---|---|---|
| | | | | | | 16:0 | 16:1 | 18:1 |
| Newborn | 45 | 45.9 | 1.03 | 1.28 | 20.6 × 10⁷ | 38.6 | 15.9 | 33.4 |
| Six months | 60 | 27.2 | 0.59 | 0.63 | 10.1 × 10⁷ | 28.0 | 6.6 | 39.2 |
| Two and one- half to two years | 64 | 31.1 | 0.74 | | 7.9 × 10⁷ | 23.2 | 4.7 | 51.6 |

Adapted from Ref. 87

### The Suckling Period

If the mechanisms at work in adult animals are similar to those in the newborn, the changes occurring at birth are in many cases induced by the sudden change in diet, which in most mammalian species consists in a change from a high carbohydrate diet to one high in fat content (milk). The details of this change, particularly for the rat, have already been discussed (2). Weaning in the rat usually consists in a decrease in the fat content of the diet (2) (Fig. 4). In man these dietary changes are much more difficult to follow, since premature weaning is the rule and the composition of the food fed to infants is determined by the fancies, fads, and fashions current in the family and the community.

There is little doubt that the high-fat milk diet is reponsible for the sustained elevation of lipid levels in the blood and thus for the metabolic differences in lipid metabolism found between suckling animals on the one hand and fetuses and weaned animals on the other. Thus, even though the initial postnatal rise in the level of lipids in the blood may not be solely due to the feeding of milk (see p. 109), subsequent changes can be ascribed to the diet. This is well illustrated for the blood level of cholesterol in man which rises to a certain level in the newborn, even if starved, but reaches the usual higher level only if milk is fed (75). Similarly, in the suckling rabbit a high carbohydrate diet decreases the blood level of lipids (76) and in suckling rats starvation decreases the level of fatty acids in the blood (2). Starvation of newborn rats slows down the normal rise in the rate of ketone body production (5).

In this connection the gut appears of special significance. The rate of fat absorption from the intestinal tract is somewhat lower in the

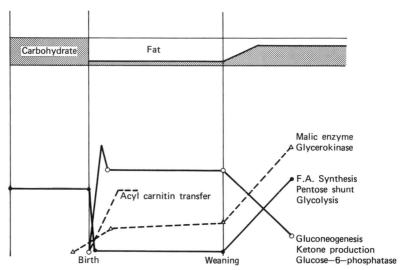

**Fig. 4.** A scheme to show the relationship between changes in diet composition and enzyme activities. The two horizontal lines at the top of the diagram indicate the composition of the diet, dotted being carbohydrate, white being fat. The space on the left represents the fetal period, the space in the middle, the suckling period, and the space on the right, the weaning and postweaning period in the rat. The changes in malic enzyme and glycerokinase activities are similar in liver and adipose tissue. Fatty acid synthesis also changes in a similar fashion in liver and adipose tissue but not brain. The pentose shunt, glycolysis, gluconeogenesis, ketone body production, and glucose-6-phosphatase are all for the liver.

newborn than about a month after birth (77). This difference is not striking and depends on the type of triglyceride contained in the diet (Fig. 5). Apparently the position of palmitate in the triglyceride molecule, for instance, is of considerable importance (78) (Table 10). It is surprising that lipase activity in both the gut, the pancreas, and the

**Table 10    Percent Absorption of Fatty Acids from Lard and Randomized Lard[a]**

|  | Palmitic Acid | Stearic Acid | Total |
|---|---|---|---|
| Lard | 94 | 88 | 95 |
| Randomized lard[b] | 58 | 40 | 72 |

[a] Adapted from Filer et al. (78).
[b] Randomized lard has 33.9% of palmitic acid in position 2 of the triglyceride; normal lard, 85.3%.

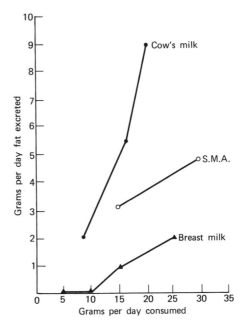

**Fig. 5.** Relationship between the amount of fat consumed and the amount of fat excreted in the stools of newborn infants. Cow's milk: a preparation based on dried cow's milk with added lactose. S.M.A.(S.M.A./S26): made from skimmed milk and a fat mixture similar in fatty acid composition to breast milk (77).

liver (Table 11) only gradually attains the adult level in rats, puppies, and man (2). An attempt was made to explain this by suggesting that triglycerides are absorbed as such to a greater extent from the gut of

**Table 11    Lipolytic Activity in Rat Organs as Percent of Adult**

|  | Fetus | Newborn | 7 Days | 25 Days | Adult | Refer- ence |
|---|---|---|---|---|---|---|
| Esterase, liver | 18 | 18 | 50 | 150 | 100 | 115 |
| Lipase, liver (microsomes) | 50 | 100 | 280 | — | 100 | 115 |
| Mitochondrial lipase, liver | 16.7 | 16.7 | 100 | — | 100 | 115 |
| Lipase, pancreas | — | 11.8 | 11.8 | 94 | 100 | 2 |
| Lipase, gut | — | 26.6 | 33.3 | 80 | 100 | 2 |

newborn rats than from that of older animals (79). Now it appears that a further mechanism might also be at work for some time after birth. As already mentioned, the rate of triglyceride synthesis in the fetal gut of sheep (Table 4) and perhaps also of man is high. After birth, before the lamb is fed, triglycerides appear in the thoracic lymph in the form of lipoproteins but not chylomicra (80), and chylormicra also appear only gradually in the blood of newborn infants (2). Thus, although lipase activity in the gut is low and the rate of fat absorption is also somewhat lower than later in life, the gut seems equipped to carry the newborn through this period by actively supplying it with fat. Hence a more detailed examination of the mechanisms of fat absorption in the newborn in the suckling period should be worthwhile. For our knowledge on this subject up to about 1966 see (2) and (81).

In rats, as would be expected, the rate of FA synthesis is high in the fetus, decreases rapidly after birth, stays low for the whole period of breast feeding, and increases again as weaning occurs (Figs. 4 and 6). Again we know nothing about these processes in human beings.

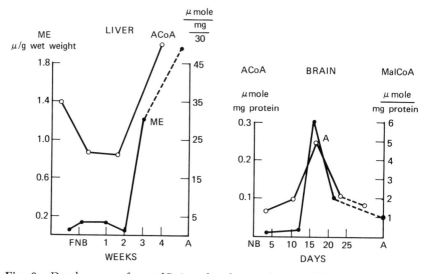

Fig. 6. Development of acetylCoA carboxylase in brain and liver, malic enzyme in liver, and fatty acid synthesis from malonylCoA in the brain. F = fetus, NB = newborn. *Left:* acetylCoA carboxylase ($\mu$mole/mg-30 min) in liver (124) and malic enzyme ($\mu$moles/g-min) in liver (13). *Right:* rate of incorporation of labeled acetylCoA or malonylCoA into fatty acids of brain microsomes (124).

A more detailed analysis of the processes concerned has been undertaken in the heart by Wittels and Bressler (7) and to a lesser extent in liver and adipose tissue by ourselves (82). In this connection it is perhaps useful to point out that it is not permissible to extrapolate from data obtained in one organ to other organs. Thus, for instance, processes in the liver change in a completely different way than processes in the brain (Fig. 6) (Table 12). This is not surprising when we consider that homeostasis in one way or another is important throughout the life of the animal. The liver is one of the organs maintaining homeostasis and so to some extent is adipose tissue. Brain, on the other hand, is

Table 12    Effects of Aceto-acetate in Rat Brain Slices

|  | 1–3 days | Adult |
|---|---|---|
| Acetoacetate $\to$ $CO_2$ as % of glucose $\to$ $CO_2$ | 200% | 60% |
| RNA biosynthesis (avidine incorporation) | 100% | 40% |
| Percent of glucose effect 7-min |  |  |
| nucleotide phosphate | 1.82 $\mu$mole/g | 1.28 $\mu$mole/g |
| + acetoacetate | 2.81 $\mu$mole/g | 1.47 $\mu$mole/g |
| + glucose | 3.07 $\mu$mole/g | 2.13 $\mu$mole/g |
| [Adapted from Itoh and Quastel (114)] |  |  |
| Percent increase in $O_2$ consumption of brain slices on addition of 60 mg % glucose to medium | +78% | +114% |
| Percent increase of same on addition of 60 mg % acetoacetate to medium | +80% | +33% |
| Utilization of glucose by brain slices: $\mu$moles/100 mg day weight/60 min | 370 | 290 |
| Utilization of acetoacetate by brain slices, $\mu$moles/100 mg day weight/60 min | 190 | 67.5 |
| Ratio of AA/glucose consumed | 0.51 | 0.23 |
| [Adapted from Drahota et al. (113)] |  |  |

an organ that requires homeostasis and is probably being protected by the organism from unnecessary tasks. Thus, although in the whole animal the rate of fatty acid synthesis is undoubtedly low in the suckling period, the rate of fatty acid synthesis in the brain and also the rate of lipid synthesis and of the laying down of lipids in that organ is probably highest in that period, at least in the rat. This, of course, is a further indication that nutritional changes have only small effects on the brain, whereas their effect on liver and white adipose tissue is much greater. Nevertheless, even the brain is indirectly affected by the high fat diet. The utilization of acetoacetate by brain slices from suckling rats is greater than later in life (Table 10), whereas glycolysis seems to be suppressed. We have suggested elsewhere (39) that in the early postnatal period of the rat ketone bodies are utilized to a

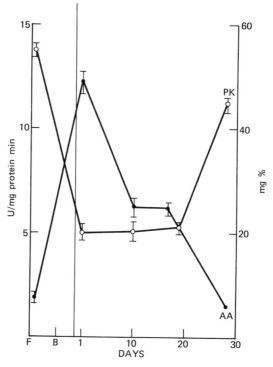

**Fig. 7.** Changes in pyruvate kinase activity in the brain of infant rats and changes in the level of acetoacetate in the blood of these same animals. PK = pyruvate kinase, AA = acetoacetic acid, F = fetus, and B = birth.

much greater extent than before birth and later in life (Fig. 7). This is indicated by the rapid rise in the blood level of these substances, by the high rate of ketone utilization in the brain and also the heart (7), and by the much slower development of carnitine-activated fatty acid oxidation in the heart (7) and thus perhaps also in other organs and tissues.

Nothing is really known in this respect about brown adipose tissue. In the liver and white and brown adipose tissue of the rat another enzyme involved in fatty acid synthesis also goes through changes that we could expect on the basis of the changes in nutrition. The synthesis of malonyl-CoA by acetyl-CoA carboxylase occurs at a much greater rate in the fetus than in the suckling animal and returns to higher levels after weaning. The same is true of the synthesis of fatty acids from both acetate and citrate but only if we consider the supernatant fraction of adipose tissue (82). This is in contrast to what is found in the liver in which both liver slices and the enzymes involved show lower activity in suckling rats (82, 83). The reasons for this are not difficult to find. Adipose tissue cells, particularly those of white adipose tissue, increase in size because they accumulate fat after birth (84) (Table 9). Hence the rate of synthesis of fatty acids in individual cells of white adipose tissue and to a lesser extent of brown adipose tissue decreases throughout life (85). The decrease during the suckling period is due to a decrease in enzyme activities and also to an increase in cell size. The decreases after weaning are due only to increasing cell size. This increase in cell size after weaning is apparently greater than the increase in enzyme activities, and the overall result is a further decline in the rate of fatty acid synthesis per one adipose tissue cell. This explains why, although enzyme activities in suckling animals are lower than in weaned animals, the rate of fatty acid synthesis per unit wet weight or per single cell of adipose tissue is greater in suckling animals than in weaned animals.

The rate at which fat is accumulated in adipose tissue after birth in the rat is high, and it is undoubtedly true that this is due not only to fatty acid synthesis in adipose tissue but more so, probably, to the laying down of fat supplied by the milk. If this is true, we would expect that the fatty acid composition of adipose tissue fat would reflect the fatty acid composition of the milk as shown in several mammalian species (86), including man (87). In this connection it is of particular interest that in the suckling period of rats the number of cells in adipose tissue is being determined by the amount of calories supplied to the animal (88). It has been shown by Hirsch and associates that underfeeding rats during the suckling period by maintaining about 13 animals with one mother results in a decreased final number of adipose tissue cells in epidydimal fat. Overfeeding suckling rats, on the other hand, by maintaining only three rats in one litter increases the final number of cells in adipose tissue. No biochemical data are available that could be correlated with these morphological alterations. Considering that even the brain itself is affected by such procedures (89, 90, 91, 92), it is too early to come to any definite conclusions. We shall return to this problem later.

What, then, do we know about the enzymatic development in liver, in white adipose tissue, and in brown adipose tissue. Table 5 surveys our present-day knowledge. In order to make the data more meaningful, we have also included some enzymes of glucose metabolism. It is apparent that delivery triggers off a number of biochemical processes and that those shown here can be explained by the sudden change in diet.

In fact, there are two sudden changes. The first change, as already mentioned, is really a temporary complete lack of food. The second change is the sudden supply of a high-fat diet (for details see Ref. 2). Since, in adult animals, the effect of starvation and a high-fat diet on enzyme activities is similar, it is not surprising that the initiation of extrauterine life, regardless of whether started by starvation or the high-fat diet, is typified by the same sort of changes. As glucose starts to be in short supply, fatty acids are being utilized. In the rat, and to a lesser extent also in man, this results in increased formation of ketone bodies by the liver (5), depression of fatty acid synthesis (83), and an initiation of gluconeogenesis (9). These processes are so intimately interwoven that it is probably useless to consider each of them entirely independently.

If we take the liver as our reference organ, the obvious effect of delivery is a depression of glycolysis and an induction of fatty acid oxidation and gluconeogenesis. All these changes can be induced in the adult animal, either by starvation or a high-fat diet. As already mentioned, it is probable that these changes are triggered by starvation, at least in man, and subsequently by the high-fat diet.

Here it is worthwhile pointing out that the same effect is achieved by starvation in man and the high-fat diet in the rat. There are two differences in this respect between man and the rat. First, man is born with a considerable amount of fat in his body, whereas the rat contains little fat, and the amount that it does contain is not present in white adipose tissue. This tissue appears only a day or two after birth. The second difference between these two species lies in the fact that although man is usually not fed at all until after the first 24 hours of life the newborn rat is suckled within about half an hour after delivery. Yet in both species the sudden changes that occur after birth are similar (at least all the evidence so far indicates this). This can be explained by the fact that in both species the level of free fatty acids in the blood increases rapidly, although for somewhat different reasons. In the rat the increase is due mainly to the early feeding of the newborn. In man, on the other hand, it is due to mobilization of fatty acids from the lipid depots. In both cases it appears that the initiators of all these enzymatic changes are (a) the increased level of free fatty acids in the blood and thus in all organs and (b) the decreased availability of glucose.

It is interesting to consider the effects of premature delivery or of intrauterine malnutrition (dysmature babies) in this connection. The level of FFA and TG in the umbilical blood of dysmature newborns is much higher than usual (94, 95) and the intravenous infusion of lipids to such newborns does not induce a rise in the level of ketones in their blood (96, 97). Thus it seems that in dysmature newborns the prolonged lack of nutrients prevents them from utilizing fatty acids either by oxidation or triglyceride synthesis to the extent that is usual in normal full-term infants. Alternatively, it might be postulated that the fatty acids are utilized so rapidly that no ketone bodies appear.

Roux (98) has shown that premature delivery in rabbits induces suppression of fatty acid synthesis in the liver and that fatty acid synthesis is still high in postmature fetuses (Table 5). Thus the moment of delivery appears decisive (for discussion see Ref. 39).

The effect of diet on metabolic development cannot be seen solely as the action of individual nutrients or their metabolic products on certain cells of various tissues. It seems that the effect of diet may be much more subtle than this, and a recent paper to that effect is worth considering in some detail (99). In adult rats the enzyme tyrosine-amino transferase can be induced in their liver by injection of cortisone or by feeding a high-protein diet. The same enzyme in late rat fetuses is inducible by glucagon, norepinephrine, or cyclic AMP but not by cortisone. A similar mechanism is at work for the induction of glucose-6-phosphatase in the fetal liver. Yet after birth the increase in the amount of this enzyme can be inhibited by feeding glucose. Hence the responsiveness to environmental changes is conditioned by

(a) the receptor sites of the enzyme (for instance) to certain agents;
(b) the presence or absence of these agents in the body (e.g., hormones);
(c) components of the diet itself.

It is quite possible that in some cases changes in diet do not act directly on, say, liver cells but indirectly by inducing or suppressing the release or formation of a hormone or even a nerve impulse. This is well illustrated in adult animals in the case of insulin which is released into the circulation in response to hypoglycaemia.

Unfortunately, as far as lipid metabolism goes our knowledge is less than fragmentary and much we are going to say here is pure speculation. The postnatal development of lipid metabolism in itself and in relation to the diet has been studied only in a few species. This is unfortunate from the point of view of nutrition, since the nutrition of different species varies considerably; for instance, the rabbit is born with little subcutaneous fat but with a large amount of brown adipose tissue. It is fed once a day by the dam and for the rest of the 24 hours goes without food. The guinea pig again starts feeding on whatever is available almost immediately after birth, as do most ruminants, even though all mammalian species also take in breast milk.

Species difference after birth are considerable so that certainly many more important relationships could be glimpsed by a comparison of these different types of development. Nevertheless, there are some factors that seem to be universally applicable to mammalian infant animals during the suckling period. They are fed primarily a high-fat diet (milk) and one in which it is impossible for them to differentiate between the intake of fluids and solids. This, of course, is not completely true of those species in which the newborn immediately consumes food other than milk, but even in these species the diet usually contains more fat than later in life. Hence we should expect it to be a universal phenomenon that the rate of lipid synthesis after birth is decreased in all mammalian species. This should be true even for such species as the guinea pig which actually loses fat during the first 10 days after birth. Such a loss of fat entails the oxidation of fatty acids and again logically would indicate a depression of fatty acid synthesis, at least in the liver and adipose tissue. This has, however, never been examined in any detail, if at all.


## Weaning

The weaning period has been shown to be considerably important to further development (for details see Ref. 2). In the rat it commences on about the fourteenth postnatal day and is terminated on about day 30, when rats no longer consume any breast milk. During these 16 days of life suckling rats gradually increase their consumption of solid food and decrease their intake of milk. As far as lipids are concerned, there is no doubt that they play an important role in that period (see next section). Premature weaning of the rat to the normal laboratory diet suddenly decreases fat intake and consequently sets off a series of events, including probably an increase in the rate of fatty acid synthesis, in the rate of glucose utilization for energy purposes, and a decrease in gluconeogenesis. A recent paper by Smith (118) gives good evidence that diet is the decisive element in fatty acid synthesis of suckling animals. Fatty acid synthetase activity decreases rapidly after birth in mice and increases again on weaning. Premature weaning leads to a premature rise in enzyme activity which can be prevented by the administration of actinomycin, indicating that the rise in activity is due to *de novo* synthesis. In addition, it has also been possible to induce fatty acid synthesis in seven-day-old mice by feeding the mothers a linoleic acid-free diet [such a diet induces fatty acid synthesis in adult mice but not rats (117)]. Other enzymes affected in a similar way but to a lesser extent are acetyl-CoA synthetase and citrate cleavage enzyme.

In this connection it is noteworthy that many functions attain a much more mature level on about day 18, including such diverse ones as thermoregulation (2), secretion of adrenal cortical hormones (2), thyroid function (100), muscle innervation (2), brain maturation (104), and enzymes in the gut (81). Most of this maturation occurs between days 14 and 18 (i.e., at a time when weaning commences). In some cases it has been possible to delay these changes by feeding a high-fat diet to the dam and her offspring. By doing this it is possible, for instance, to maintain a high blood level of ketone bodies, a level that cannot be attained by adult rats fed the same high-fat diet (103). Since adrenal cortical functions also mature between days 14 and 18, it would be interesting to know how far the diet affects these processes. Adrenalectomy performed in 14-day-old rats, for instance, will also delay the fall in the blood content of ketone bodies, though no such effect is seen in adult animals (103).

In man the weaning period is badly defined and much too little is known about the effects of premature weaning, particularly in Western society, in which this occurs frequently within a week after birth. The so-called humanized milks now used contain a large amount of unsaturated fatty acids, and there are some indications that the infants fed these formulas require more Vitamin E than a breast-fed infant (104). An infant fed cow's milk, on the other hand, may be receiving a less-than-adequate supply of unsaturated and essential fatty acids. The differences between various milk formulas are well discussed by Straub et al. (105) and (106) and the importance of breast milk is stressed by Davies (107). Figure 5 shows that the rate of fat absorption also depends on the type of milk given to the infant and underlines our lack of knowledge in this area.

## Late Effects of Nutritional Alterations Early in Life

Several years ago it seemed a logical but by no means obvious assumption that environmental changes occurring early in life are more effective than those occurring later during development in altering the organism (2). As mentioned at the beginning of this chapter, development is not a smooth ascending and descending curve. It is now fashionable to talk about critical periods* of development, and this term implies that sudden changes are seen at certain stages of the life-span. It also implies that it is more probable that the environment will channel further development along specific lines during these critical periods of development than at other times. It is perhaps worthwhile to point out that similar ideas have been with us for some time, starting probably with the early Darwinians in Russia: Timiryazeff and Mitchurin. The man who made a caricature of these ideas was, of course, Lysenko. It appears that we are going to rediscover many such thoughts now, but we should be very careful with our conclusions. The general subject has been discussed repeatedly. Here we should like to point out that a thorough understanding of the mechanisms involved in such late effects of early environmental changes can be obtained only by understanding the developmental processes themselves. It seems likely that critical periods of development in the same individual differ for different tissues and even cells, since development of the body is not a uniform process. There are many indications that show differences in enzyme development in liver, kidney, brain, and so on. Morphologically this has been obvious for a long time (a budding limb can be deformed, a completed limb is unaffected). Biochemically, we know little in that respect. As far as lipids go, it might be worthwhile to look into the possibility of early nutrition affecting subsequent development in the following areas.

### Atherosclerosis

It was first suggested by Gillman and Gillman (108) that the roots of adult human atherosclerosis should be sought in early infancy. The only evidence to date comes from our data showing that early weaning of rats to a normal diet makes them more susceptible to an atherogenic diet when aged 8 months (2). Nothing more is known in this field and most certainly further research should uncover many new facets.

---

* There are two ways of defining a critical period. One is to define it by the consequences of environmental changes at that time. Thus we might say that the early postnatal period in the rat is a critical period, since overnutrition at that time (or for that matter undernutrition) leads to permanent changes later in life. Another way of defining a critical period is more exact. It considers the mechanisms responsible for a certain period being critical. From that point of view a critical period is a certain interval during the development of an animal when certain events in certain cells occur for the first time. Such events might be differentiation, cell division, or a sudden rise or decrease in certain enzyme activities. It is most important here to keep an open mind, since it is easy to confuse the issue by giving labels to badly understood processes, prematurely. This is exactly what Lysenko did when he defined critical periods of development.

## Obesity

Here we are on firmer ground. It has been shown that early overfeeding leads to an increased number of adipose tissue cells (88) later in life, to increased fat content in the body, and thus to overweight (88). Alternatively, depending on your point of view, underfeeding in infants causes lower adult body weight, adipose tissue contains fewer cells, and the body has less fat. Thus the quantity of food consumed by the rat in early postnatal life determines its final body weight (109, 110), probably by determining the final number of adipose tissue cells in its body. It would be interesting to confront these data with earlier work which demonstrated that underfeeding prolonged the life-span of rats (111). In that work, however, underfeeding was initiated after weaning, and there are no data on animals underfed from the moment of birth or even in utero as far as longevity goes.

There are some indications that the fat infant will also be the obese adult, even in man.

## Mental Ability and Conditioned Reflexes

Prematurely weaned rats when adult (one year) have a poor memory (a conditioned reflex is more easily extinguished) and poorer learning capacity (the conditioned reflex takes longer to be elaborated) when compared with normally weaned animals. These effects or premature weaning can be nullified by feeding a high-fat diet between days 18 and 30 after birth (2). Evidently the fat in the diet is important for further development of the brain in the weaning period.

## Sexual Development

Prematurely weaned male rats when aged 6 months or 1 year show degeneration of the testes. This is particularly marked in animals prematurely weaned to a high-carbohydrate diet. This premature degeneration of the testes can be completely prevented by feeding the prematurely weaned rats a high-fat diet (2).

## CONCLUSIONS

In most mammals three nutritional periods can be distinguished during their development:

1. High-carbohydrate nutrition during fetal life
2. High-fat nutrition during suckling
3. Adult diet after weaning

Metabolic processes reflect these nutritional characteristics.

1. In the fetal period glucose utilization prevails. Fatty acids are synthetized.

2. In the suckling period glucose is in short supply and fatty acids are utilized to a greater extent.

3. After weaning metabolic processes adapt to the prevailing adult diet.

A change in the quantity or quality of the diet during development may have far-reaching consequences more pronounced than those resulting from a change in diet in adult animals.

The following references are review articles and may be helpful to the reader in becoming acquainted with more details of work in this field: 2, 3, 20, 33, 39, 53, 108, 124, 125, 126, 129.

## REFERENCES

1. F. B. Stifel, N. S. Rosenzweig, D. Zakim, and R. H. Herman, *Biochim. Biophys. Acta* **170**: 221 (1968).

2. P. Hahn and O. Koldovsky, *Int. Ser. Monographs in Pure and Applied Biology*, Vol. 33. Oxford: Pergamon.

3. E. W. Page, *Amer. J. Obstet. Gynecol.*, **104**: 378 (1969).

4. P. Hahn, E. Vavrouskova, J. Jirasek, and J. Uher, *Biol. Neonat.* **7**: 348 (1964).

5. Z. Drahota, P. Hahn, A. Kleinzeller, and A. Kostolanska, *Biochem. J.* **93**: 61 (1964).

6. F. Sauer and J. D. Erfle, *J. Biol. Chem.* **241**: 30 (1966).

7. B. Wittels and R. Bressler, *J. Clin. Invest.* **44**: 1639 (1965).

8. P. C. Greenfield and E. J. Boell, *J. Exptl. Zool.* **168**: 491 (1968).

9. F. J. Ballard and R. W. Hanson, *Biochem. J.* **104**: 866 (1967).

10. H. B. Burch, O. H. Lowry, A. M. Kuhlman, C. Skerjance, E. J. Diamant, S. R. Lowry, and P. Dippe, *J. Biol. Chem.* **238**: 2267 (1963).

11. P. Hahn and R. Greenberg, *Experientia* **24**: 928 (1968).

12. F. J. Ballard and I. T. Oliver, *Biochem. J.* **95**: 191 (1965).

13. R. W. Hanson and F. J. Ballard, *Biochem. J.* **108**: 705 (1968).

14. L. N. Fain and R. O. Scow, *Amer. J. Physiol.* **210**: 19 (1966).

15. J. F. Roux, A. Grigorian, and Y. Takeda, *Nature* **216**: 819 (1967).

16. J. F. Roux, *Biol. Neonat.* **13**: 109 (1968).

17. G. Popjak and M. L. Beeckmans, *Biochem. J.* **46**: 547 (1950).

18. C. A. Villee in *Physiology of Prematurity*, 2nd Macy Foundation Conf. (1958).

19. P. Hahn and Z. Drahota, *Experientia* **22**: 706 (1966).

20. E. M. Widdowson, *Proc. Nutr. Soc.*, **28**: 17 (1968).

21. M. Dobiasova, P. Hahn, and O. Koldovsky, *Biochim. Biophys. Acta* **70**: 713 (1963).

22. C. A. Villee and D. D. Hagerman, *Amer. J. Physiol.*, **194**: 457 (1958).

23. Z. Koren and E. Shafrin, *Proc. Soc. Exptl. Biol. Med.* **116**: 411 (1964).

24. C. M. Van Dayne, R. J. Havel, and J. M. Felts, *Amer. J. Obstet. Gynecol.* **84**: 1064 (1962).

25. M. S. Hershfield and A. M. Nemeth, *J. Lipid Res.* **9**: 460 (1968).

26. C. M. Van Duyne, R. H. Parker, R. J. Havel, and L. W. Holm, *Amer. J. Physiol.* **199**: 987 (1960).

27. A. J. Szabo, R. D. Grimaldi, and W. F. Jung, *Metabolism* **18**: 406 (1969).

28. O. W. Portman, R. E. Behrman, and P. Soltys, *Amer. J. Physiol.* **216**: 143 (1969).

29. A. F. Robertson and H. Sprecher, *A. Ped. Scand.* **183**: 3 (1968).

30. B. L. Walker, *Lipids* **2**: 497 (1967).

31. V. Sabata, H. Wolf, and S. Lausmann, *Biol. Neonat.* **13**: 7 (1968).

32. M. Novak, V. Melichar, and P. Hahn, *Biol. Neonat.* **7**: 179 (1964).

33. V. Sabata, P. Hahn, and Z. Drahota, *Exc. Med. Monogr. Symp. Prague* **140** (1966).

34. R. O. Scow, S. S. Chernick, and M. S. Brinley, *Amer. J. Physiol.* **206**: 796 (1964).

35. D. P. Alexander, H. G. Britton, N. M. Cohen, and D. A. Nixon, *Biol. Neonat.* **17**: 178 (1969).

36. A. F. Robertson, H. Sprecher, and C. Dobbs, *Biol. Neonat.* **14**: 32 (1969).

37. W. E. Connor and D. S. Linn, *J. Lipid Res.* **8**: 558 (1967).

38. V. Sabata and M. Novak, *Gynaecologia* **163**: 179 (1967).

39. P. Hahn.

40. L. Picon, *J. Physiol.* **60**: 275 (1968).

41. A. Jahn, U. Joppe, L. Winkler, and E. Goetze, *Acta Biol. Med. German* **19**: 231 (1967).

42. V. Sabata, Z. K. S. Stembera, and M. Novak, *Biol. Neonat.* **12**: 194 (1968).

43. P. Hahn and R. Greenberg, *Life Sciences* **7**: 187 (1968).

44. P. Hahn and J. Skala, *Biol. Neonat.* (in press).

45. C. Garbarsch, *Histochemie* **18**: 168 (1969).

46. H. M. Cunningham and W. M. F. Leat, *Canad. J. Biochem.* **47**: 1013 (1969).

47. J. J. Biezenski, *Amer. J. Obstet. Gynecol.* **104**: 1177 (1969).

48. P. A. Weinhold, *Biochim. Biophys. Acta* **187**: 85 (1969).

49. J. Baldwin and W. E. Cornatzer, *Lipids* **3**: 361 (1968).

50. M. Dobiasova and P. Hahn, *Physiol. Bohemoslov.* **17**: 26 (1968).

51. T. Fujiwara and F. H. Adams, *Proc. Soc. Exptl. Biol Med.* **128**: 88 (1968).

52. T. Fujiwara, F. H. Adams, S. Sipos, and A. El-Salawy, *Amer. J. Physiol.* **215**: 375 (1968).

53. M. Cornblatt and R. Schwartz, in *Major Problems in Clinical Pediatrics.* Saunders, 1966.

54. M. J. Dawkins, *Brit. Med. Bull.* **22**: 27 (1966).

55. M. Coquoin-Carnot and J. M. Roux, *C. R. Soc. Biol.* **156**: 442 (1962).

56. G. Guroff and C. A. Rhoads, *J. Neurochem.* **16**: 1543 (1969).

57. M. Novak, V. Melichar, P. Hahn, and O. Koldovsky, *Physiol. Bohemoslov.* **10**: 488 (1961).

58. C. M. Van Duyne and R. J. Havel, *Proc. Soc. Exptl. Biol. Med.* **199**: 757 (1959).

59. M. J. Hardman and D. Hull, *J. Physiol.* **201**: 685 (1969).

60. M. J. Hardman, E. N. Hey, and D. Hull, *J. Physiol.* **205**: 51 (1969).

61. M. J. Hardman, E. N. Hey, and D. Hull, *J. Physiol.* **205**: 39 (1969).

62. G. Alexander and S. C. Mills, *Biol. Neonat.* **13**: 53 (1968).

63. V. Melichar and H. Wolf, *Klin. Wochenschrift* **46**: 549 (1968).

64. T. Heim and D. Hull, *J. Physiol.* **187**: 271 (1966).

65. C. T. Gurson and L. Etili, *Arch. Dis. Child.* **43**: 679 (1958).

66. P. Hahn, M. Novak, and V. Melichar, *Physiol. Bohemoslov.* **15**: 493 (1966).

67. M. Novak, V. Melichar, and P. Hahn, *Biol. Neonat.* **9**: 105 (1965/1966).

68. M. Novak, P. Hahn, and V. Melichar, *Biol. Neonat.* **14**: 203 (1969).

69. R. E. Smith and B. A. Horwitz, *Physiol. Rev.* **49**: 330 (1969).

70. R. F. Dyer, *Amer. J. Anat.* **123**: 255 (1968).

71. N. Mrosovsky and U. Rowlatt, *Biol. Neonat.* **13**: 230 (1968).

72. M. J. R. Dawkins and J. W. Scopes, *Nature* **206**: 201 (1965).

73. J. I. Pedersen, E. N. Christiansen, and H. J. Grav, *Biochem. Biophys. Res. Commun.* **32**: 492 (1968).

74. K. J. Hittleman, O. Lindberg, and B. Cannon, *Europ. J. Biochem.* **11**: 183 (1969).

75. R. Kohn, M. Novak, M. Melichar, M. Havlova, and M. Vinsova, *Čs. pediat.* **16**: 979 (1961).

76. M. Friedman and S. O. Byers, *Amer. J. Physiol.* **201**: 611 (1966).

77. D. A. T. Southgate, E. M. Widdowson, B. J. Smith, W. T. Cooke, C. H. M. Walker, and N. P. Mathers, *Lancet* **487**: 489 (1969).

78. L. J. Filer, Jr., F. H. Mattson, and S. J. Fomin, *J. Nutr.* **99**: 293 (1969).

79. O. Koldovsky, P. Hahn, V. Melichar, M. Novak, P. Prochazka, J. Rokos, and Z. Vacek, *Biochim. Biophys. Library* **1**: 161 (1963).

80. A. D. Shannon and A. K. Lascelles, *Austr. J. Biol. Sci.* **22**: 189 (1969).

81. O. Koldovsky, *Development of the Functions of the Small Intestine in Mammals and Man.* Basel: Karger, 1969.

82. P. Hahn, *Physiol. Bohemoslov.* **19**: 369 (1970).

83. K. K. Carrol, *Canad. J. Biochem.* **42**: 83 (1964).

84. J. Hirsch, and P. W. Han, *J. Lipid Res.* **10**: 77 (1969).

85. P. Hahn, R. Greenberg, M. Dobiasova, and Z. Drahota, *Canad. J. Biochem.* **46**: 735 (1968).

86. K. Bernhard and H. Bodun, *Helv. Chim. Acta* **29**: 1782 (1946).

87. G. L. Baker, *Amer. J. Clin. Nutr.* **22**: 829 (1969).

88. J. L. Knittle and J. Hirsch, *J. Clin. Invest.* **47**: 2091 (1968).

89. M. Winick, *J. Pediat.* **74**: 667 (1969).

90. M. A. Fishman, A. L. Prensky, and P. R. Dodge, *Nature* **221**: 552 (1969).

91. W. J. Culley and R. O. Lineberger, *J. Nutr.* **96**: 375 (1968).

92. H. P. Chase, W. F. B. Lindsley, Jr., and D. O'Brien, *Nature* **221**: 554 (1969).

93. M. L. Brown and H. A. Guthrie, *Growth* **32**: 143 (1968).

94. V. Šabata, K. Znamenacek, H. Pribylova, and V. Melichar, *Symp. Prague*, **435** (1966).

95. V. Šabata and Z. K. Stembera, *Exc. Med. Mon. Symp. Prague*, **561** (1966).

96. V. Melichar, Kreislauf-und Stoffwechsel-probleme bei Neubeborenen u. Sauglin-gen, S. Melsungen, **126** (1968).

97. V. Melichar, Fortschritte der parenteralen Ernahrung Pallas Verlag, Lochham bei Munchen, **125** (1967).

98. J. Roux, *Metabolism* **15**: 856 (1966).

99. O. Greengard, *Biochem. J.* **115**: 19 (1969).

100. F. A. Hommes, C. W. Wilmink, and A. Richters, *Biol. Neonat.* **14**: 69 (1969).

101. R. Balazs, B. W. L. Brooksbank, A. N. Davison, J. T. Eayrs, and D. A. Wilson, *Brain Res.* **15**: 219 (1969).

102. L. Krawiec, C. A. G. Argiz, C. J. Gomez, and J. M. Pasquini, *Brain Res.* **15**: 209 (1969).

103. P. Hahn, Z. Drahota, and O. Koldovsky, *Experientia* **20**: 625 (1964).

104. S. A. Hasim and R. H. Asfour, *Amer. Clin. Nutr.* **21**: 7 (1968).

105. C. P. Straub, *J. Amer. Diet. Assoc.* **54**: 381 (1969).

106. Committee on Nutrition, *Pediat.* **26**: 1039 (1960).

107. P. A. Davies, *Proc. Nutr. Soc.* **28**: 66 (1969).

108. J. Gillman and T. Gillman, *Perspectives in Human Nutrition.* New York: Green & Stratton, 1951.

109. A. S. Parkes, *Ann. Appl. Biol.* **13**: 374 (1926).

110. G. C. Kennedy, *J. Endocrinol.* **15**: 19 (1957).

111. C. M. McCay, L. A. Maynard, G. Sperling, and L. L. Barnes, *J. Nutr.* **18**: 1 (1939).

112. H. Wolf, V. Melichar, and R. Michaelis, *Biol. Neonat.* **12**: 162 (1967).

113. Z. Drahota, P. Hahn, J. Mourek, and M. Trojanova, *Physiol. Bohemoslov.* **12**: 134 (1965).

114. T. Itoh and J. H. Quastel, *Proc. Canad. Fed. Biol. Soc.* **11**: 88 (1968).

115. P. Hahn, A. Drahota, and M. Novak, *Biol. Neonat.* **9**: 82 (1965/1966).

116. W. S. Schwark and D. J. Ecobichon, *Biochem. Farmac.* **18**: 915 (1969).

117. J. R. Sabine, H. McGrath, and S. Abraham, *J. Nutr.* **98**: 312 (1969).

118. S. Smith and S. Abraham, *Arch. Biochem. Biophys.* **136**: 112 (1970).

119. P. Hahn, J. Skala, K. Vizek, and M. Novak, *Physiol. Bohemoslov.* **14**: 546 (1965).

121. J. Skala, T. Barnard, and O. Lindberg, *Comp. Biochem. Physiol.* **33**: 509 (1970).

120. T. Barnard, J. Skala, and O. Lindberg, *Comp. Biochem. Physiol.* **33**: 499 (1970).

122. P. Hahn and J. Skala, *Comp. Biochem. Physiol.* **41B**: 147 (1972).

123. E. Aeberhard, J. Grippo, and J. H. Menkes, *Pediat. Res.* 3: 590 (1969).

124. "Foetal Autonomy," G. E. W. Wostenholme and M. O'Connor, Eds. *CIBA FDTN Symp.*, London: Churchill, 1969.

125. T. Barnard and J. Skala, in *Brown Adipose Tissue*, O. Lindberg, Ed. New York: Elsevier, 1970.

126. G. S. Dawes, *Foetal and Neonatal Physiology*. Chicago: Year Book Medical Publishers, 1968.

127. Z. Drahota, E. Honova, and P. Hahn, *Experientia* **24**: 431 (1968).

128. J. Skala and O. Lindberg, *Intern. J. Biochem.* **1**: 513 (1970).

129. Development of Metabolism as Related to Nutrition, P. Hahn and O. Koldovsky, Eds. Basel: Karger, 1966.

# 5

# Hormonal and Dietary Factors in the Development of Digestion and Absorption

O. KOLDOVSKÝ

Division of Biochemical Development and Molecular Diseases, Children's Hospital of Philadelphia and Department of Pediatrics, Medical School of the University of Pennsylvania, Philadelphia

All nutrients that enter the body must first pass through the gastrointestinal tract. Hence the functioning of this organ is of vital significance to the proper functioning of the body as a whole. For these reasons it is important to understand the factors that influence the development of the gastrointestinal tract.

The action of this organ during development is in part a response to changes in diet. Although the food of adult animals may be characterized as a high-carbohydrate, low-fat diet, maternal milk in almost all species is a high-fat, low-carbohydrate diet (108) (Fig. 1). Not only does the fat content of milk differ from that of the adult diet, but differences also exist in the carbohydrate composition (lactose versus starch), dietary proteins (casein versus heterologous proteins), and minerals.

Although, as with other organs, it is important to attempt to correlate gastrointestinal function with structure, in this chapter we deal mainly with changes in the physiology and biochemistry of digestion and absorption. There are several reviews of the development of the gastrointestinal tract structure (69, 70, 170, 171, 334).

Studies of the development of the gastrointestinal tract have been viewed with increased interest during later years. We discuss mainly the newer publications; the older literature can be found either in my reviews (170, 171) or in recently published reviews from other laboratories (69, 131, 244).

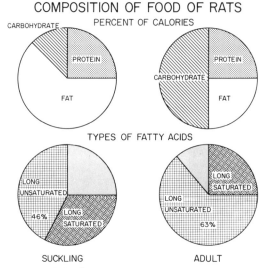

**Fig. 1.** Composition of food of suckling (milk) and adult rats. (*Upper*). Caloric percentage of fat, protein and carbohydrates. Data taken from (108) (*Lower*). Percentage of different fatty acids of the lipids in food. Dotted: 10:0, 12:0, 14:1; cross-hatched: long saturated, 16:0, 18:0. Hatched: long, unsaturated: 18:1, 18:2, 18:3, 20:4. From (73).

## MOTOR ACTIVITY OF THE GASTROINTESTINAL TRACT

### Swallowing

Swallowing appears in mammals as early as the fetal period in rabbits and monkeys (21, 40), sheep (259), and guinea pigs (24). The human fetus starts to swallow amniotic fluid between the third and fifth month (66, 223, 279). Contrast material injected into the amniotic sac appears sooner in the stomachs of older fetuses than in those of younger ones. As prenatal development progresses, the rate of gastric emptying increases and the material moves more rapidly along the small intestine. Thus certain constituents of amniotic fluid might be broken down and absorbed from the fetal gastrointestinal tract.

### Evacuation of the Stomach

Evacuation is slower in suckling rats than in adults (25, 127, 296). Emptying of glucose from the stomach is controlled by osmoreceptors present in the duodenum. Husband and Husband (150) have shown that these osmoreceptors are already functioning in babies during the first few days of life, since a solution containing a higher glucose concentration (10%) left the stomach more slowly than a 5% solution. Since polysaccharides are poorly digested by infants, a 10% starch solution leaves the stomach more rapidly than a 10% glucose solution. By contrast in adults these isocaloric solutions empty at the same rate (151).

## Automatic (Rhythmic) Movements of the Small Intestine

These movements appear in guinea pig fetuses together with the appearance of Auerbach's plexus. Koshtoyants and Mitropolitanskaya (192) observed spontaneous rhythmic activity of the small intestine in human fetuses as early as six to seven weeks. This activity also correlates with the appearance of Auerbach's plexus. The same authors (193) also reported that rhythmic activity increases with age. Windle and Bishop (347) and Ehrhardt (81) have described the presence of peristaltic movements in 3- to 5-month-old human fetuses. Acetylcholine causes a prompt contraction of human fetal ileum in vitro (34). Epinephrine, isoprenoline, or norepinephrine relaxed this contraction and their effects did not change in fetuses between 11 and 23 weeks of age (224). Koshtoyants (191), summarizing his experiments published during the thirties, showed that the distal part of the small intestine in infant rabbits does not show automatic motor activity during the suckling period. This activity appears only at the time of weaning.

## Movement Along the Digestive Tract

The propulsive mobility of the gastrointestinal tract accelerates with age during fetal life [guinea pigs (24), rhesus monkeys (305), human fetuses (223)], and further postnatally [lambs (48), rats (176, 296), and man (298)]. In piglets no change in the rate of passage of food along the whole gastrointestinal tract was noted between 6 days and 17 days of age (166).

In contrast, passage through the large intestine decelerates with age; for example, emptying of the large intestine was most rapid in premature infants (162), less rapid in full-term infants, and slowest in older infants (298). A similar inverse relationship with age has been described in rats (296).

## CARBOHYDRATE DIGESTION AND ABSORPTION

### Digestion of Polysaccharides

Amylase appears *prenatally* in the pancreas of horses, cows (3), and sheep (163). In man pancreatic amylase is not consistently present at birth (164, 169).

Amylase was detected by Auricchio et al. (11) in the small intestine of a 3-month-old fetus.

Amylase activity increases postnatally in dogs and rats and shows a marked increase at weaning (Fig. 2) (274). In man amylase activity has been reported to be absent or low in the intestinal content of infants of less than 6 to 12 months of age (7, 12, 35, 105, 106, 169). In agreement with these results a lower degree of polymerization of carbohydrates was found in duodenal juice in children younger than 6 months than in children 1 to 2 years old (12).

## Digestion of Disaccharides

### Lactose

$\beta$-Galactosidase exists in at least two multiple forms (9). One of the isoenzymes is localized in the microvilli of the enterocytes (4, 182) together with other disaccharidases (58, 59). If other characteristics are used for identification, this enzyme appears to correspond to what is commonly called "lactase." The other isoenzyme is localized in the lysosomes (4) and has been called either "acid" $\beta$-galactosidase or hetero-$\beta$-galactosidase. Here we discuss the first isoenzyme; the latter is described later.

The presence of lactase in the intestinal mucosa has been proved in many mammals. Only the California sea lion and Steller's sea lion (310) have no disaccharidase activity in the small intestine. Their milk does not contain lactose. Lactase was found prenatally in pigs (336), rabbits (74), and man (11, 64, 317). In human fetuses activity of lactase does not change between 11 and 23 weeks of embryonic life (64). It increases before birth both in man (11) and in rabbits (74). After birth the activity decreases; its decrease may be related to the stage of maturity as determined by the length of the suckling period. In guinea pigs weaning begins on the day of birth, and in this species lactase activity decreases least (68).

In man it was found that lactase activity in the mucosa of the small intestine is higher in term newborns than in adults (11). This finding is not in full agreement with the data of Boellner et al. (30). In the cat the decline in activity occurred most rapidly at 4 to 7 weeks of age, which again coincides with the weaning period in this animal. Changes in the rat were studied by several authors (74, 147, 282). Because acid $\beta$-galactosidase activity interferes in the assay of the activity of neutral $\beta$-galactosidase (lactase), in this species a method was developed for the specific determination of neutral $\beta$-galactosidase by using the fact that $p$-chloromercuriobenzoate inhibits the activity of the

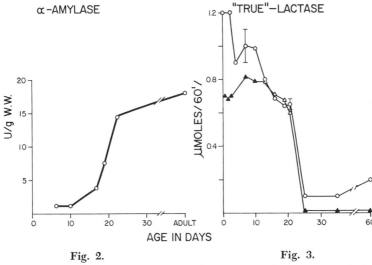

Fig. 2.                                   Fig. 3.

**Fig. 2.** α-Amylase activity in pancreatic homogenates during postnatal development of the rat. S.E. smaller than circles. Ordinate: activity in units per g wet weight of pancreas (278).

**Fig. 3.** Postnatal development of neutral β-galactosidase ("true" lactase) in rat jejunum (○) and ileum (△). Mean values are presented; vertical lines denote 2 × S.E.M. Full symbols denote that the difference between the values for the jejunum and ileum of that particular age group is statistically significant (P < 0.01) (189).

acid β-galactosidase but has no effect on the activity of the neutral β-galactosidase (186).

With this method it was found (Fig. 3) that the activity in both jejunum and ileum was greater in the suckling period than in later life. Between day 20 and day 25 after birth the activity in both areas fell rapidly to reach adult values. The difference in the activity of the neutral β-galactosidase between the jejunum and ileum was greatest in adult animals, in which the ileal activity represented about 20% of the jejunal activity; the difference was also marked in the newborn period, but there was no difference in activity in 12- to 20-day-old rats. From that we might speculate that the digestion of lactose occurs along the entire length of the small intestine during the suckling period, whereas in the new-born and adult animals the digestion of lactose is more restricted to the upper portions of the small intestine (247).

### Other Disaccharides

We again restrict our description to a few selected species; for details see Koldovský (170). Tachibana (315, 316) has demonstrated the presence of maltase and sucrase in the human small intestine during the first months of embryonic life. Tachibana and Fomina (95) also observed an increase of sucrase in the third month.

The development of disaccharidases in human fetuses has been studied in recent years by several authors (11, 64, 157) (Fig. 4b). Most of

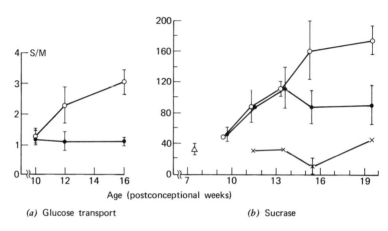

*(a)* Glucose transport                    *(b)* Sucrase

Fig. 4.    Development of glucose absorption and sucrose activity in human fetuses. (*Left*). Ratio of glucose concentration in serosal fluid (S) to that in mucosal fluid (M) in jejunum (○) and ileum (●) of human fetuses. Ordinate: S/M ratio. Abscissa: age in postconceptional weeks. Vertical lines denote 2 S.E.M. (156). (*Right*). sucrose activity of the jejunum (○), ileum (●), and colon (X) of human fetuses of different ages. Activity is given as milligrams of reducing substances liberated from 5.5% sucrose solution at pH 6.25/60 min/g w.w. Small vertical lines denote 2 S.E. small intestine not separated in the jejunum and ileum. Abscissa: age in postconceptional weeks (157).

the α-glucosidase activities (maltase, sucrase, isomaltase, palatinase, and trehalase) reach a maximum between the sixth and eighth months of gestation (11). Dahlqvist and Lindberg (64) studied fetuses 11 to 23 weeks old and found no change in maltase and isomaltase activities within this period. Enzyme activities were approximately 50% of those found in adults. Total maltase activity of fetuses differs further from that in adults, since maltase II and III (defined by heat inactivation) are absent in human fetuses. These maltases develop later in gestation. In newborn infants the mucosa of the small intestine has the same activity of sucrase, isomaltase, and total maltases as the mucosa of adults (11). In different animals the maltase, isomaltase, sucrase, and trehalase activities are low but increase during the weaning period (Fig. 5).

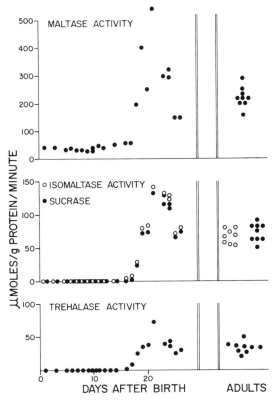

**Fig. 5.** Activity of disaccharides in the small intestine of rats of various ages (282).

## Absorption

### *Disaccharides*

*Sucrose.* The low sucrase activity in suckling animals correlates well with the slow rate of disappearance of sucrose from the gastrointestinal tract of 1-week-old piglets compared with 3-week-old piglets (167).

*Lactose.* In good agreement with the findings of high lactase activity in the suckling period lactose absorption is higher both in suckling rats (184) and in newborn rabbits (309). In chicken Boellner et al. (30) determined the blood sugar after oral lactose application. Immediately after birth absorption of lactose from the gastrointestinal tract is slow, as indicated by the small and slow increase in blood sugar, compared with changes in blood sugar after a glucose load. Within the first 14 days of life the difference in blood glucose increase after the oral administration of lactose or glucose disappears.

### Monosaccharides

*Active transport of hexoses* was demonstrated during gestation in rabbit (71, 346), guinea pig (45), pig (44), rat (46), and man (181). In animals the rate of transport increases before birth. In man (156) it increases only in the jejunum, leading to a jejunoileal difference (Fig. 4a). This active transport of hexoses has several characteristics similar to those .found in adults; i.e., it is inhibited by phlorizin (71) and the increase of the transmural potential difference (208), but it differs by being independent of oxygen supply as it is in adults [animals (71, 346) and human fetuses (156, 208)]. This shows that anaerobic processes supply sufficient energy for active transport mechanisms in the fetal small intestine.

What does the existence of active transport in the fetal small intestine mean? Two main explanations are possible:

1. It has no functional significance, being only the first appearance of a mechanism that will become important at the beginning of oral nutrition.

2. Since the fetus swallows amniotic fluid, it is possible that hexoses and amino acids can become substrates for active transport.

Both McLain (223) and Mengert and Bourland (228) suppose that the gastrointestinal tract can take part in regulating the amount and composition of amniotic fluids in humans.

Postnatally the state of maturity influences the absorption of glucose. This absorption proceeds at a slower rate in premature babies than in term newborns (35). In guinea pigs (born mature) active transport of α-methylglucoside decreases during the first week of postnatal life, whereas the absorption of glucose increases postnatally in mice (46) and rats (91, 173).

### Other Sugars

The introduction of *fructose* into the lumen of the small intestine of sheep fetuses in a concentration higher than the level of fructose in fetal plasma is followed by an increase of fructose in fetal blood (249, 349). In 1- to 3-week-old pigs *fructose* and *xylose* disappeared from the lumen of the gastrointestinal tract more slowly than glucose. The low rate of fructose removal could be related to the very low activity of fructokinase in the intestinal wall of young pigs (1).

# PROTEIN DIGESTION AND ABSORPTION

## Digestion

### Role of the Stomach

*Gastric secretion* has been studied prenatally in many species, but only data obtained in rat, guinea pig, and man are discussed here. [For further details see Vollrath (333), Koldovský (170), and Deren (70).] At birth the gastric content of the rat has a pH of 5.0 to 6.6 (124, 125, 140, 218). Just before birth the guinea pig fetus shows spontaneous secretion of an acid gastric juice (311). Between the forty-seventh and fifty-fifth day of gestation the pH of the gastric content is 7.0 to 8.0. In 68-day-old fetuses a pH of 4.0 was measured.

Postnatally the acidity of the stomach contents increases in all species studied. This increase can be correlated with mucosal maturity as assessed by anatomical appearance. In guinea pigs the pH of the gastric content drops to adult values immediately after birth. In both untreated (140, 218) and histamine-stimulated (124, 125) rats the pH of the gastric content decreases with maturity. By 10 days histamine-stimulated rats reach values close to values found in adult animals. These values are attained by the fourth week of postnatal life without stimulation (218). By determining carbonic anhydrase activity it has been concluded that hydrocholoric acid secretion begins on the second postnatal day in both rats and guinea pigs (333). Quantitative determinations made by Helander (124, 125) confirm this finding and show a further 50% increase between 10-day-old and adult rats.

The pH of gastric fluid in newborn infants is usually neutral or slightly acid (149), but after birth the gastric pH decreases rapidly (79, 119, 149). In newborns with high birth weights the free acidity of the gastric content is said to be higher than in newborns with low birth weights (231); furthermore, children born with low birth weights showed achlorhydria more frequently than children born with high birth weights (230). This finding, however, was not confirmed by Harries and Fraser (119), Thomson (320), or Ames (6). Secretion of free acid is considerably lower in premature than in full-term infants after a meal or after histamine administration (231). The actual pH of the stomach contents in infants depends strongly on food intake as shown by Mason (220), who measured pH of the gastric content of infants 5 to 13 days old during feeding. He found that the entry of milk into the infants' stomach causes a sharp increase in the pH (Fig. 6). Total gastric acidity, which

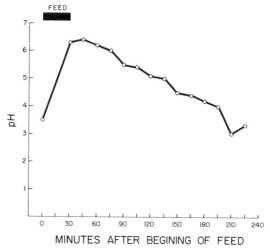

Fig. 6.   Mean values of pH of the stomach contents of 25 newborn infants during the intervals between feeds. [Children were fed at the breast at approximately four-hour intervals (220).]

increases during postnatal life, shows its most rapid rise during the first three months and then levels off at the end of the first year (231).

Proteolytic activity was found in the stomachs of rat fetuses three days before birth (about 10% of activity of adult rats) (124, 125). There is approximately a threefold increase in this activity during the last three days of embryonic life. In human fetuses older than 16 weeks proteolytic activity in the stomach was described by Keene and Hewer (164). According to Wagner (335), the production of proteolytic activity begins in the fundus during the third month. In the antrum secretion is minimal. Pepsinogen is excreted by the kidneys into the amniotic fluid and appears between the seventh and eighth month of gestation.

Postnatally, activity in the stomach of newborn and suckling rats is low; the proteolytic activity is several times higher in rats aged 21 to 35 days (29, 245). Helander's data (124, 125) also show an increase between 10-day-old rats and adults, but the activity doubles only between these two developmental stages. Milk-clotting activity of the rat stomach homogenates increases before birth and is almost constant during the suckling period. In adults this activity is as low as in fetuses (124, 125). The peptic activity of the stomach of newborn infants is proportional to the degree of maturity (340); e.g., in newborns of 4000 g it is about four times higher than in prematures weighing 1000 g. Proteolytic activity in the fundus increases about four times after food intake on the second day of postnatal life (335). Mason (220) found no substantial digestion of protein in specimens of gastric contents taken from 5- to 8-day-old infants. A most probable explanation for this finding is that the pepsin is almost completely inactivated at the high levels of pH that were found in the stomach at various intervals after feeding. In older infants (13 to 44 days; mean 23 days of age) (26) traces of hydrolyzed protein were found in stomach contents, cows' milk proteins being hydrolyzed to a higher degree than the proteins of human milk.

### Role of the Pancreas

In the pancreas the activity of trypsin increases during gestation in sheep (163), in calves, (148, 286), and in human fetuses. The pancreatic proteolytic enzymes begin to form within the third month of human gestation; at that time typical granules can be detected in the pancreas (164). Similar results were obtained by Fomina (95), Tachibana (318), and Blum et al. (28). Permanent secretion starts at the beginning of the fifth month.

Trypsinogen and chymotrypsinogen were found in the pancreas of fetuses of more than 500 g (209). The activity did not increase before birth, and low values were measured only in fetuses weighing 350 to 500 g. These results are in contrast to those of Werner (340) who, using histological and biochemical methods, found low proteolytic activity (activated by enterokinase) in infants with low birth weights. In prematures of less than 1000 g no granules were found; in infants with birthweights between 1000 and 2000 g granules appeared rarely; and in full-term babies granules were numerous. The proteolytic activity in newborn infants of 4000 g was found to be about six times higher than in infants weighing 1000 g. Gschwind (105) made a similar observation but did not use the method of activation with enterokinase.

Enterokinase appears in fetuses weighing 390 g (153). According to Lieberman (209), activation of trypsinogen by pancreatic tissue occurs only in fetuses weighing 1500 g or more. The discrepancy between the data of these authors might be due to different analytical methods and procedures for obtaining and storing material; both authors used samples from stillborn infants.

The proteolytic activity of the homogenates of the pancreas increases after birth in calves (mainly during the first week of life) (148), pigs (about the fifth week of life) (120), and rats (between the fourth and sixth postnatal week) (146).

Trypsin activity in duodenal juice of 1-week-old premature infants was described to be lower than in 2- to 4-week-old infants. Food intake did not increase the trypsin excretion in those infants (35). According to several reports, the trypsin and chymotrypsin activities do not change substantially after birth in full-term infants during several years of life (7, 106, 217). In the Hadorn et al. (106) study the authors compared both the concentration and the total ouput per kilogram of body weight of trypsin and chymotrypsin in infants and did not find differences between different age groups (0–6, 6–12 months and 1–5, 5–13 years of age).

### Role of the Small Intestine

*Proteases* were investigated during the prenatal period only in human fetuses. Keene and Hewer (164) demonstrated "erepsin" activity in fetuses 16 weeks old and Tachibana (312) found "erepsin" activity in 3-month-old fetuses. Protease activity in the jejunum did not change markedly between the eighth and the seventeenth weeks of gestation, but in the ileum a pronounced increase was found (133).

Postnatally, studies ave been performed on pigs and rats. It was found that the proteolytic activity in the small intestine of newborn piglets is low and that it increases during the first two postnatal months (120). Several protein-hydrolyzing enzymes in rats have been studied (170, 250). Chymotrypsin activity increases before weaning and does not change later on. Trypsin activity could be detected only in the ileal mucosa of suckling rats. It disappears after weaning. This activity originates most probably from pancreatic trypsin that has been absorbed, from the lumen, by ileal enterocytes, since after 24 hours of starvation the activity in the lumen is reduced to one-tenth and no more activity can be detected in ileal homogenates. Proteolytic activity decreases during postnatal development.

During incubation of everted sacs of the small intestine from fetal and newborn pigs no degradation of albumin was found; in sacs from 1- to 7-day-old pigs part of the recovered albumin was found to be degraded (44). Its origin (whether from the small intestine or from the pancreas) was not studied.

*Peptidases* were studied in different animals and different substrates were used. Since only a few peptidases have been defined, their nomenclature often relies on the identification of the substrates used. Their localization in the cell (i.e., whether in microvilli or in other cell particles) is often an open question, and for many of them it also remains to be elucidated whether these enzymes are actively involved in digestion of food or whether they are only part of the cell metabolism of the enterocytes.

Various peptides have been split by preparations of the fetal small intestine of the rat (212), guinea pig (53), pig (211), and man (28, 133, 210, 283). Prenatally peptidase activities increase in the rat [substrates: glycyl-valine, glycyl-leucine, glycyl-glycine, alanyl-glutamate, and alanyl-proline (212)] and the pig [alanyl-glutamic acid, alanyl-proline, and glycyl-leucine (211)]. Gamma-glutamyl transpeptidase (53) decreases by one order of magnitude during the last week of pregnancy in guinea pigs. In human fetuses Blum et al. (28) noted an increase of splitting in glycyl-glycine in the third month of gestation, whereas Lindberg (212), confirming the presence of this dipeptidase and demonstrating several others (see Table 1, p. 168) in the small intestine of fetuses aged 11 to 23 weeks, did not observe any pronounced developmental changes. A similar amount of dipeptidase activities was observed in the large intestine (210). Heringova et al. (133), measuring aminopeptidase activity with leucyl-$\beta$-naphthylamid as substrate in human fetuses, saw no change of activity in the jejunum between the eighth and seventeenth weeks after conception but did see an increase in the ileum. Tripeptidase activity (glycyl-glycine as the substrate) changed only slightly in the same period. The homogenates of the small intestine of human fetuses also split glutamyl-proline and glycyl-proline. No substantial changes in the activities of these peptidases were observed after the sixteenth week of age. The levels of both enzymes were comparable with those of adults (283). Although optimum pH and Km of glycyl-proline dipeptidase did not change during the age period studied, glutamyl-proline dipeptidase of 14- to 24-week-old fetuses displayed a different pH optimum and different $Km$ than later.

Postnatally peptidase activities increase in the guinea pig [gamma-glutamyltranspeptidase (53)]. Lindberg and Karlsson (211) observed a postnatal decrease of dipeptidase splitting glycyl-leucine and alanyl-glutamic acid in pigs, whereas no postnatal change of activity was observed with alanyl-proline as substrate. In rats, according to Heizer and Laster (123), the alanine-phenylalanine hydrolase activity increases postnatally with a spurt between day 15 and day 25. Further, in rat it was found that the postnatal development of tripeptidase, aminopeptidase activity, and dipeptidase (glycyl-glycine) is similar (170, 250). Increases of activity of the jejunum occurred at the time of weaning, but no substantial changes were observed in the ileum. Further, dipeptidase activities have been determined in the rat—with glycyl-valine, glycyl-leucine, glycyl-glycine and alanyl-glutamate as substrates—by Lindberg and Owman (212). Shortly after birth these activities increase to adult levels, whereas analyl-proline hydrolase activity does not increase before weaning. Lindberg and Karlsson (211) have shown an interesting effect of colostrum intake on dipeptidase activities of the small intestine of the pig. They have found that in newborn pigs fed by colostrum dipeptidase splitting glycyl-leucine and alanyl-glutamic acid decreases to 50% of the values for unsuckled animals.

## Absorption of Proteins and Their Breakdown Products

### Absorption of Intact Proteins

The absorption of intact protein by the immature mammalian gastrointestinal tract varies with the species and with the stage of ontogeny.

In our review we discuss this question briefly for several reasons. The problem has been studied mainly by immunologists because the transfer of intact antibodies in colostrum and milk plays an important role in immunological reactions of newborn animals. Reviews by Brambell (36), Morris (244), and Koldovský (170) and Brambell's (37) recently published book devoted to this topic enable the interested reader to get a detailed picture elsewhere.

We now discuss briefly several aspects of the subject: the existence and duration of transfer of intact proteins in different mammals through the gastrointestinal tract, the mechanism(s) conditioning the transfer of proteins across the wall of the gastrointestinal tract of infant mammals, the location of transfer of intact proteins along the length of the small intestine, the route of transfer of absorbed proteins from the small intestine, and factors affecting the cessation of transfer of intact proteins.

*The Existence and Duration of Absorption of Intact Proteins.* This subject may be divided into two main questions. First, what type of protein is absorbed by the small intestine, and, second, in what animals and when in the perinatal period does this absorption of intact proteins occur?

Most information is available on antibody absorption (37, 244). Some other studies deal with the absorption of insulin in different species (165, 245, 269), lactate dehydrogenase (16), albumin (44, 50, 86, 159, 270, 271), and ferritin (195) or a macromolecular substance such as polyvinylpyrrolidine (51, 52, 115, 116, 202) or colloidal gold (50).

Intact protein absorption has been observed *prenatally* in guinea pigs (205) and rats (39), but in fetal rabbits no transfer of protein across the intestinal wall could be detected (38). *Postnatally* intact proteins are transferred for a few days in piglets, calves, goats, horses, and cats. In puppies proteins pass through the intestinal wall for about one week (221, 228, 288); in rats and mice during the first three weeks of life [Halliday (109) and many others], and in hedgehogs for as long as six weeks (243). No transfer of proteins in the gastrointestinal tract could be detected in guinea pigs and rabbits after birth (37). In humans the data are conflicting. Brambell (37), reviewing the literature, shows that most papers deny the possibility of transfer of passive immunity after birth. Studies by Leissring, Anderson, and Smith (206), on the other hand, show the existence of this transfer. Brambell (37) asks for confirmation of these results. He concludes this part of his review with this statement:

There is no reason to doubt that very small amounts of intact proteins, including immune globulins, may be transmitted from the gut to the circulation of the newborn infant, as they can be in the adult . . . for it is well known that people can be anaphylactically sensitized by proteins absorbed by the alimentary tract. The weight of evidence at present is against the transmission of passive immunity to the circulation of the human infant after birth.

Insulin has a hypoglycemic effect after oral application but only up to 20 minutes after birth; later it has no effect on the blood glucose level (351).

*The Mechanism(s) Conditioning the Transfer of Proteins Across the Wall of the Gastrointestinal Tract of Infant Mammals.* Two important factors seem to condition the existence of intact protein transfer. The first is proteases of the gastrointestinal tract and the second is peculiarities of the small intestine. The low activity of pepsin and low acidity of the gastric contents in newborn suckling mammals coincide with the period of intact protein absorption. Although a difference of magnitude of one order was found in proteolytic activity and pH of the stomach content in suckling mammals in comparison with adult individuals, no similar differences in proteolytic and peptidase activities have been described for the small intestine. The absence of protein hydrolysis in the stomach seems to be more decisive than the difference in similar processes in the small intestine. The effect of orally administered insulin- on blood glucose levels demonstrates the importance of gastric digestion. When insulin is administered perorally in rats, it causes a decrease of blood sugar only in the suckling period (245). On the other hand, when it is applied directly into the small intestine *in situ*, it causes a decrease in blood sugar level in both suckling and weaned rats (Hiršová and Koldovský, unpublished). Further, the finding of no difference between the effect of introjejunal and introileal administration in infant rats, although there is a multiple difference in the proteolytic activity of the two parts of the small intestine (250), suggests that this proteolytic activity does not interfere substantially in the process of insulin absorption.

Some breakdown of gamma-globulin occurs, nevertheless, in newborn animals, also after oral administration, although a substantial part passes intact into the peripheral circulation. Hardy (117) found that the degree of hydrolysis was higher in pigs 15 to 20 hours old than in those less than five hours after birth.

Further, the small intestine possesses other peculiarities that account for intact protein transfer.

Although chronologically information about intact protein absorption was obtained first in experiments in vivo, we begin with experiments in vitro.

Studies were performed on rats by Nathan (246), Bamford (20), and Rodewald (277); pigs were studied by Lecce (200), Pierce and Smith (270, 271), Smith and Pierce (299), and Brown, Smith, and Witty (44).

Slices from the small intestine of newborn and 5-day-old piglets accumulate pig gamma-globulin. Similar slices from adult mice and rabbits do not possess this quality (200). This process requires sodium and is inhibited by metabolic inhibitors [iodoacetate, arsenate, fluoride, 4,6-dinitro cresol, phlorizin, Lecce (200); NaCN, Bamford (20)]. Albumin is transferred by everted intestines of pigs more readily than gamma-globulin (270, 271); rat gamma-globulin is transported faster than bovine or rabbit gamma-globulin (20). Transport of albumin increases the oxygen consumption of the everted sac of the rat's small intestine in vitro (20). Brown et al. (44) also have shown a relation between albumin and sodium transport. Bovine lactoglobulin transport is inhibited by l-leucine and l-methionine; l-alanine and d-isomers of these aminoacides have no effect (299) and poly-l-arginine increases this transport, whereas poly-l-glutamic acid alone has no effect. However, addition of this last to poly-l-arginine abolishes the stimulatory effect of poly-l-arginine (300).

In vivo experiments have shown that absorption of intact protein is dependent on the dose in rats (111) and pigs (270), and some proteins are absorbed faster and to a greater extent than others. This phenomenon of selectivity has been analyzed (42, 113, 242). Recently Jordan and Morgan (159) have shown that the selectivity might change also with age in rats. Absorption of albumin ceased first, then of $\alpha$-globulin, finally of $\beta$- and gamma-globulins. In mice (241) and rats (41, 111), a so-called interference was found during antibody absorption; i.e., antibody absorption is decreased in the presence of another immunoprotein or even another protein to a higher extent than could be explained by dilution only. Absorption of gamma-globulin [and polyvinylpyrrolidone of mean molecular weight 160,000 (115, 116)] is accelerated in newborn pigs

(116) and newborn calves (18, 115) by factors present in the colostrum. In pig these factors are heat labile, whereas in the calf they are heat stabile. In calves substantial stimulation is obtained by lactate, pyruvate, and salts of lower volatile fatty acids. These active compounds, however, are not found in colostrum in significant quantities. It is interesting that intravenous infusion of $l$-lactate facilitates the absorption of polyvinylpyrrolidone (mol wt 160,000) introduced into the duodenum in water. This indicates that some of the solvent factors that accelerate absorption may reach the lower intestinal segment, in which the absorption occurs, via the blood vascular system after they have been absorbed from the upper small intestine. Electron microscopic studies (50) on mice and rats, demonstrate that proteins enter the cell by pinocytosis, i.e., invagination of the apical membrane. Using cytochemical, immunological, and electronmicroscopic methods, Graney (101), Wissig and Graney (348), Kraehenbuhl and Campiche (196), Cornell and Padykula (56, 57), and Rodewald (277) described in detail the processes that occur during the protein absorption at the cellular level, especially the function of the "apical endocytic complex."

*Location of Transfer of Protein Along the Length of the Small Intestine.* The data on protein transfer do not agree on which part of the small intestine is more important for this process. Only the duodenum is excluded. Histologically, protein transfer was observed both in the jejunum and in the ileum [Clark (50) in rats and mice]. Some authors studied mainly the jejunum (83, 196, 277, 322) and found that section important. On the other hand, the existence of large vacuoles in the enterocytes of the ileum in suckling animals observed by Smith (302), Comline, Roberts, and Titschen (54, 55) in calves, Wissig and Graney (348), Clarke and Hardy (51, 52) in rats, and Leissring and Anderson (205) in guinea pigs led these authors to stress the ileum as the location of intact protein absorption.

To document this open question I have selected several figures from different papers. The first are from experiments on rats (Fig. 7); the others (Fig. 8) are from experiments on pigs. The accumulation of macromolecular polyvinylpyrrolidone (which is not transported from the gut of rat) takes place predominantly in the distal protions, after oral administration. Rodewald's (277) results show that more antiferrin (differences of five twofold dilutions) appears in the peripheral circulation if applied to the ligated proximal rather than to the distal segment of the small intestine. Finally, a third possibility is offered (i.e., no difference between jejunum and ileum): application of insulin via the same route as in Rodewald's experiments causes a similar decrease of blood sugar levels (Hiršová and Koldovský, unpublished), whether ap-

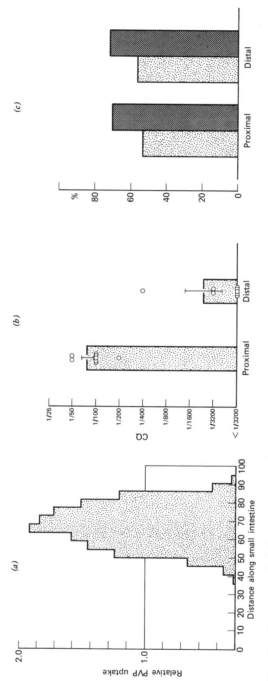

**Fig. 7.** Absorption of different proteins along the length of the small intestine of the suckling rat. (*a*) The longitudinal distribution of ($^{125}$I)PVP recovered from the wall of the small intestine four hours after feeding. Rat 16 days old. Ordinate: relative ($^{125}$I)PVP uptake. Abscissa: distance along small intestine 0 = pylorus; 100 = ileo-caecal valve. Uniform and total uptake of all PVP passing the pylorus would be represented by the area enclosed by the rectangle (51). (*b*) Comparison of antiferritin titers present in the circulation one hour after injection of antiferritin immunoglobulin into the proximal or distal ligated segment of the small intestine. CQ equals antiferritin titer in the serum divided by antiferritin titer in the injected immunoglobulin. Circles show values for individual animals. Bars and vertical lines show means and standard errors, respectively (277). (*c*) Comparison of blood glucose levels one hour after application of insulin (60 IU/100 g b.w. = □ or 6 IU/100 g b.w. ■ ) into the proximal or distal ligated third of the small intestine. Given as the percentage of the level found in rats in which 0.9% NaCl was applied instead of insulin [Hiršová and Koldovský in (170)].

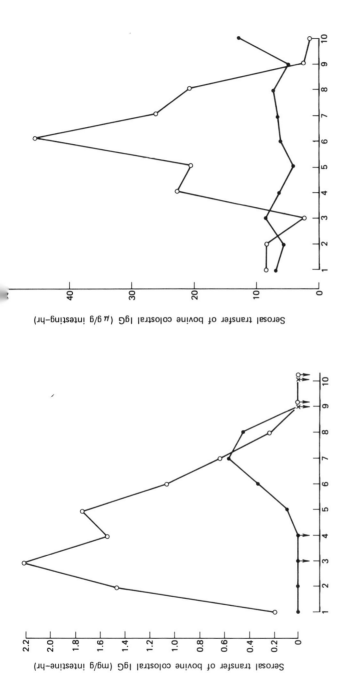

**Fig. 8.** Absorption of protein in vitro from different segments of the small intestine of newborn pig. (*a*) Serosal transfer of bovine colostral IgG by everted sacs of intestine taken from newborn pigs after feeding 2·1 ml/100 g body weight of bovine colostrum, dialyzed previously against bicarbonate saline and containing bovine colostral IgG 9·7 g/100 ml. (—○—) and 1·5 g/100 ml (—●—). The intestines were removed from the pigs 90 min after feeding and were then everted and incubated for two hours at 37°C in bicarbonate saline. Arrows show less than figures. (*b*) Serosal transfer of bovine colostral IgG by everted sacs of pig intestine. Intestines were taken from pigs shortly after birth before they had sucked the sow. Everted sacs were incubated for two hours at 37°C in various solutions of bovine colostrum previously dialyzed against bicarbonate saline containing different amounts of bovine colostral IgG. —○—, and —●— show serosal transfers of colostral IgG by sacs incubated in colostrum containing, respectively, 9·7 and 1·5 g IgG/100 ml. Slightly modified from (270).

153

plied in the proximal or the distal loop. Experiments performed in vitro on pigs by Pierce and Smith (271) are interesting from several points of view (Fig. 8). Immune lactoglobulin (271), newborn pig albumin (44), and bovine colostrol IgG are transferred maximally in the middle portion of the jejunoileum in everted sacs of unfed newborn pigs. These findings occurred only at high concentration of protein in the incubation medium. A lower concentration shows no substantial difference along the length of the jejunoileum. In contrast, if IgG is administered in vivo and transfer is then determined in vitro, we see a substantial change of pattern. A lower dose shows maximal transfer (release) in the distal portion, whereas the higher one shows a dominant transfer in the proximal portion.

It seems that the capacity of the small intestine during the suckling period to transfer intact proteins (and macromolecules) is generally a property of the entire jejunoileum but that several other factors, such as interference of other molecules, type of protein molecule, way of application, species, and probably also age of the animal (see Clarke and Hardy, 52) must be taken into consideration before the question of the relative importance of different sections of jejunoileum will finally be solved.

*The Route of Transfer of Absorbed Proteins from the Small Intestine.* The transfer of absorbed protein from cells of the small intestine into the lymph has been shown histologically by various authors (54, 55, 84, 141). On the other hand, no evidence was found by Graney (101) of the transfer of ferritin or by Kraehenbuhl and Campiche (196) of antiperoxidase and antiferritin antibodies with similar morphological methods. Direct determination of the absorbed protein concentration in the lymph and in peripheral blood showed that proteins with large molecules are absorbed mainly into the lymph, such as lactoglobulin in calves (17, 18, 268). Albumin was found in both lymph and peripheral blood (17, 18, 84, 86, 294). Proteins of small molecular weight are transferred into the blood; e.g., insulin (269).

*Factors Affecting the Cessation of Transfer of Intact Proteins.* The cessation of absorption of intact proteins in untreated animals is related to cessation of generation of cells of the "younger" type. Both in rats (50, 52) and in calves (El-Nageh, 82) it was observed that in the critical period the cells of the lower portion lose the ability to absorb intact protein first, whereas the cells of the upper portion of the villus still accumulate immunochemically detectable protein; later, as a new generation of cells reaches the top of the villus, no more protein absorption is detected at all. The "closure" caused by intake of colostrum or of some of its components in pigs and calves is probably caused by different processes that require further studies [e.g., see Hardy (115, 116), Payne and Marsh (262)].

## Absorption of Products of Protein in Breakdown

### Balance Studies

Most studies have been performed in man and farm animals to evaluate the utilization of different dietary mixtures. As mentioned in the section on fat absorption, changes in the proportion of diet components are immediately connected with changes in many other relations between food components. For this reason such experiments are difficult to compare.

According to Lloyd and McCay (214), puppies are less able to digest crude protein in a low-protein diet than young or adult dogs. Hogue et at. (145) found that protein digestibility in calves was increased at 16 weeks, compared with 7 weeks of age.

Lloyd et al. (214) studied the digestibility of protein in 3- and 7-week-old pigs. The apparent digestion coefficient increased slightly with age but it was statistically significant from 85.3 to 88.5%. Padaliková (258) investigated the absorption of proteins from a semisynthetic diet in pigs during the first month of life and found the same values in 6-, 11-, 16-, 21-, and 26-day-old pigs.

In man proteins are well retained, as shown by Feinsteine and Smith (93) for premature newborns and by direct determination of absorption by Borgström et al. (35). Other studies that deal with this problem are discussed and referred to by Widdowson (342), Zoula et al. (352), and by Southgate et al. (304).

### Absorption of Amino Acids

Most of the studies mentioned in this section employed in vitro techniques (everted sacs or accumulation into the segments of the small intestine). These methods bring definitively valuable results, but we recommend a careful approach in evaluating quantitative differences observed during development, since it has been shown that the size of the tissue fragments plays an important role in the rate of accumulation in adult animals [see Koldovský (170), p. 65].

Active transport of amino acids by the small intestine was found to be present prenatally in rabbit (71, 346), guinea pig (45), and man (208). Both in rabbit (71) and in guinea pig fetuses (45) the capacity to transport $N,N$-dimethylglycine actively appears later than the active transport of other amino acids studied ($l$-proline, glycine, $l$-valine, lysine, and methionine). In the last prenatal week the rate of accumulation increases in a nearly parallel manner for all amino acids studied in guinea pigs; in the first three weeks after birth it decreases toward adult values (45). In the rat, born less mature, accumulation of proline increases during the first three days after birth by one order of magnitude (23). The values for 3- to 4-day-old rats do not differ substantially from values obtained in 31-day-old rats. Valine is accumulated faster in slices of the small intestine from 2-day-old rats than from adults (276). The transport of this amino acid across the everted sac of the small intestine was found to be highest in 4-week-old rats and decreases thereafter with age (248). In rat changes in cystine accumulation in small intestinal slices during postnatal development show a different developmental pattern than the amino acids mentioned before. The rate of accumulation was found to be the same in newborn, 10- to 15-day-old, and adult rats, whereas in 7- and 25-day-old animals it was 60% higher (307). Several investigators have further characterized the active transport processes during development. Altogether the rate (V max) differs during ontogeny, *Km* values for valine (276) and cystine transport (307) do not differ, thus indicating a change in the number of transport sites rather than a difference in binding by the carrier(s). The transport mechanisms for amino acids in the small intestine of newborn and suckling animals are less sensitive to lack of oxygen (as is also the case in monosaccharide accumulation). Postnatally, small intestine *l*-histidine in rabbit can be transported under anaerobic conditions (346) only during the first two days of life. States and Segal (307) have shown that although anaerobiosis completely inhibits cystine accumulation in the intestine of adult rats, under similar conditions the accumulation of cystine in the small intestine of 7-day-old rats is preserved (although at only one-third the rate compared with aerobic conditions).

## LIPID DIGESTION AND ABSORPTION

### Digestion

Lipase (used here in a very broad sense) is lower in the *lumen of the small intestine* of suckling mammals compared with adults [dogs, Kryutschkova (197), rats, Rokos et al. (278)]. Duodenal fluid of human infants shows lower lipase activity shortly after birth than later (77, 92). Lipase activity was found to be lower in premature babies than in full-term infants. Hadorn et al., (106) found no differences between children 0 to 13 years of age.

Pancreatic homogenates show low lipase activity prenatally in different species [sheep, Kapralova (163), rat, Verne et al. (329), human fetuses,

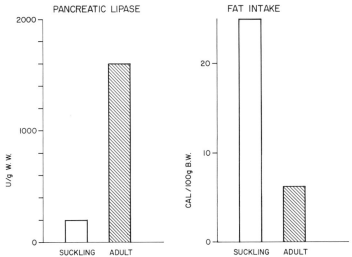

**Fig. 9.** Activity of pancreatic lipase (*left*) and fat intake (*right*) of suckling (□) and adult (■) rats. Activity given as units per g w.w. of pancreas. Fat intake is given as calories per 100 g b.w./24 hr. Data from (278) and (108).

Tachibana (313), Keene and Hewer (164)]. The activity is lower in newborn dogs (Kryutschkova, 197) and rats (Rokos et al., 278) (Fig. 9). In the rat it increases toward adult values during weaning (between the third and fourth postnatal week). On the other hand, in pigs no change of activity of lipase was observed during the first six weeks of life (168).

Small intestinal homogenates from suckling rats have a low lipase activity which increases again during weaning (278). A similar development was observed for the nonspecific esterase of the small intestine (see Fig. 14) (265) and colon in rat (219). These changes in enzyme activity seem to be in substantial contrast with the amount of fat intake, which is higher during the suckling period than later in life (Fig. 1). Perhaps further studies will supply the explanation of this paradox. At the moment we want only to stress that the type of fat consumed differs at different times. The suckling rat consumes "milk" fat; later in life, after weaning, usually fat of another origin (margarine, etc.) is supplied. Hence the fatty acid composition of these fats differs (for illustration see Fig. 1).

## Bile Acids

The bile acids play an important role in fat absorption [emulgation, micellar formation; see Hofmann and Borgstrom (143, 144)]. There have been several studies in which changes in amount, characteristics, and absorption of bile acid were determined in developing mammals. The concentration of bile acids in the duodenal juice of premature babies is lower than in full-term infants (77). Their concentration was found to increase postnatally, both in humans (31, 77, 273) and in sheep (266). The data from experiments with sheep (in which gallbladder bile was used) and the determination of bile acids in children (analysis of duodenal juice) by Poley et al. (273) show a common developmental pattern. In babies, coincidentally with the initiation of milk feeding, a sharp increase in bile acids is observed. The proportion of individual bile acids changes in the total bile during development. In infants cholic acid was the predominant bile acid (31, 273). Glycodeoxycholic acid was detected in children 15 months old and older (31, 273). Encrantz and Sjovall (87) and Poley et al. (273) have shown that the tauric conjugates exceed glycoconjugates at birth, that glycine conjugates rapidly increase within a few days after birth, and that the ratio of total trihydorxyacids to dihydroxyacids decreases with age. It is interesting also that the changes in the biliary acid pattern observed with development in sheep (266) are extremely close to those in man. Conjugation with taurine markedly exceeded that with glycine, but the amount of glycine conjugates increased with age. Glycodeoxycholic acid was not found during the first five days of life. After that time it increased until the fifth to sixth month. The first significant increase of glycoacids is seen in 1- to 2-month-old animals when milk is being replaced by a vegetable diet.

Absorption of bile acids ($^{14}$C taurocholate) has been demonstrated in dog fetuses. These data, together with previous studies of bile acid excretion by fetal liver and bile acid concentration by fetal gallbladder, demonstrate the existence of a fetal enterohepatic circulation of bile salts (297).

## Absorption of Lipids

Different criteria have been used for measuring fat absorption. The determination of the difference between the amount of fat administered orally and the amount found in the gastrointestinal tract after a given period of time yields exact results. This procedure can be applied in experimental animals as well as in human infants by using a special system of tubes. Another approach is based on the determination of fat retention (i.e., the amount of fat found in the feces subtracted from the amount of fat administered orally). Fat in the stools, however, can originate either from exogenous fat or from endogenous sources; the intestinal mucosa excretes some lipids into the lumen and this is not known to be fully independent of the amount of fat administered. Hence we have to differentiate absorption and retention.

Piglets less than 1 month old have a lower fat retention than 2-month-old piglets (61, 213). Weanling rats which are 30 to 42 days old absorb more olive oil than 6-month-old rats (72, 174).

Various studies in infants have shown that more fat is retained from breast milk than from any other food (227, 255, 304). The retention of fat from breast milk is in the range of 85 to 90%, while only 70% of cows' milk fat is retained (77, 326). The retention of heterologous fat reaches a value of 90% in about the tenth week of life. Artificially composed milk ("humanized" types) showed higher fat retention than cows' milk (304, 352).

Luther and Schreier (216) studied the absorption of stearic, oleic, and linoleic acids and olive oil in infants aged 1 to 2 months and older children. Using a balance technique for determining the retention of these fatty acids, the authors found that unsaturated fatty acids (i.e., oleic and linoleic acid) are better retained than the saturated acid (i.e., stearic acid). It is interesting to note that olive-oil retention was considerably higher, whereas 30% of the amount of stearic acid administered was lost in the stool (compared with 25% of oleic and linoleic acid and only 3% of olive oil). These results indicate that fat retention increases postnatally and that fecal losses of fatty acids in children aged 3 to 7 weeks were, on the average, higher than in children aged 10 to 17 weeks. Although the number of infants used in that study was small, the difference in oleic acid retention is remarkable.

An analysis of the ratio of individual fatty acids in breast milk and in the stool of newborn infants by gas-liquid chromatography revealed that stearic acid was absorbed to an extent of 75%, palmitic acid, 83%, and short-chain fatty acids more than 90%. The total rate of absorption of fatty acid was 85% (338).

## Lipids in the Wall of the Gastrointestinal Tract

Fat droplets were found histologically in the mucosa of the *gastric fundus* of newborn mice, but not in adults (323) Schmidt (287) did not find them in the stomach of a human fetus (8.7 cm long). Whether this variability is caused by species differences or by differences in developmental stage, we do not know. In the *colon* lipid droplets were detected both in human fetuses (2.8 to 18.0 cm long) (98, 99) and in rats after birth (99). Authors suggest that lipid absorption may take place also in a given postnatal period in this part of the gastrointestinal tube. The wall of the *small intestine* of human fetuses contains, according to Garbarsch (98), a small amount of lipid droplets in the jejunum. In fed suckling rats many more fat droplets are found than in adult animals (325). During starvation these fat droplets disappear and after refeeding (olive oil, suckling) they appear again. The relation to the food intake is further seen in results of studies in which the fat deposited in the wall of the small intestine was further characterized. Although both in pig embryos (190) and in newborn, not suckled rats (73) phospholipids only are found, a large number of triglycerides appear in the wall of the rat intestine after the first milk intake (73).

Gas liquid chromatography has further shown that triglycerides in the wall of the small intestine contain a relatively high amount of medium-chain fatty acids; in the adult rat intestine more long-chain fatty acids are present (73) which could be related to the composition of fatty acids in rat milk and the diet of adult rats.

Thus the high fat intake in the suckling period coincides with the high amount of fat in the wall of the small intestine and its lipid composition. Neutral fat might enter the intestinal mucosa cells by pynocytosis which has been observed in suckling mice and rats (50), but the neutral fat in enterocytes could also be newly synthesized from fatty acids. Reesterification of fatty acids occurs in the intestinal wall of newborn rats and dogs (175), and phospholipids are formed in the wall of the small intestine during the suckling period of rats (176, 177). According to Cunningham and Leat (62), the total glyceride synthesis (monoglyceride and $\alpha$-glycerophosphate pathways) is higher in the small intestine of sheep fetuses than after birth.

### Transport of Absorbed Fat from the Small Intestine

It is known from studies in adults that fat is transported from the gastrointestinal tract via two main routes: the lymphatic system and the portal vein. There has been no investigation of the difference between the two transport routes in newborn animals. Shannon and Lascelles (292, 293, 294, 295) have studied the composition and output of lymph in the thoracic duct of calves and have found that the concentration of lipids in lymph collected before the first feeding was high. Triglycerides comprised more than 50% of this lipid and 25% were phospholipids. Despite the very high output of triglyceride, there was no visual evidence of chylomicrons. After the first feeding the composition of the lymph lipids changes. The relative proportions of phospholipids, free fatty acids, and total cholesterol decrease, whereas the proportion of triglycerides increases. Chylomicrons in that time appeared transitory in the lymph.

During fat absorption in newborn rats and dogs (177) and infants (226) no increase in the blood level of esterified fatty acids has been observed, but the level of free fatty acids increased. In infants (226) no chylomicrons were observed in the peripheral blood during the first four to five postnatal days. The typical turbidity and increase of esterified fatty acids were found in children older than one week. As in infants, so also in rats and dogs; the increase in esterified fatty acids after fat load occurred several days after birth (176). Whether these last-mentioned phenomena are related to the absorption process or whether they are more a reflection of fat uptake and utilization by the whole organism remains an open question.

## ABSORPTION OF OTHER MATERIAL FROM THE GASTROINTESTINAL TRACT

*Water* absorption from the gastrointestinal tract increases during the postnatal development of the rat (89, 126). The increase is related to an increased rate of emptying of the stomach (25, 127).

### Absorption of Minerals

*Sodium* is actively transported by the small and large intestines of fetal sheep (349) and pigs (44).

*Magnesium* absorption proceeds more rapidly in young calves than in older animals (301).

*Calcium* transport (studied in vitro) is low in the first two weeks of postnatal life of rats and increases in the ileum markedly and progressively from two to four or five weeks (23) (Fig. 10).

Calcium retention* (studied in vivo) is higher in 14- to 18-day-old rats than in 6- to 8-week-olds (97% versus 63% of administered dose) (319). Retention of calcium was not found to be influenced by an increase in the phosphate content of the artificial milk fed to 5-day-old rats (194).

---

* When interpreting the results of retention experiments performed on suckling rats, the possible effect of recirculation of the substance studied must be taken into consideration. As Sámel and Čaputa (285) have shown with [131]I, this mineral is excreted into the urine after its application to the suckling rat. Since the suckling rat has no interoceptive micturition reflex (47), the mother licking the anogenital area removes the urine. The [131]I is then secreted into the milk and reaches the sucklings again.

*Barium, strontium, and radium* are also retained in higher amounts in 14- to 18-day-old rats than in 6- to 8-week-old rats (85, 95, 79% against 7, 25, 11% of administered dose) as found by Taylor et al. (319).

*Sulfate* accumulation (studied in vitro) is low in the intestine of suckling rats and increases several times in the duodenum during the third postnatal week (22) (Fig. 10*b*).

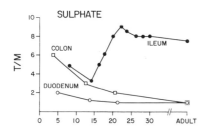

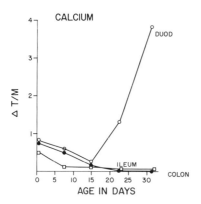

Fig. 10. Accumulation of sulfate (*upper*) and calcium (*lower*) by slices of different parts of the intestines of rats of various ages. Abscissa: age in days. Ordinate of upper part = $T/M$ (ratio of concentrations in tissue water to concentration in medium after incubation). Ordinate of lower part = difference between $T/M$ of samples incubated with inhibitors (iodo-acetate plus 2, 4 DNP) and without. ○ = duodenum, ● = ileum, □ = colon. Constructed from data given by (22, 23).

*Copper* is retained (in vivo studies) more in suckling than in weaned rats (233). Although rats retain different percentages of the metals applied in different forms (11% from biliary form, 20% from protein-bound form, and 40% from ionic form), suckling rats retain approximately 90% of all of them. Authors conclude from this and other experiments that in suckling rats more copper is absorbed and less excreted into the bile. After weaning more of this metal is excreted in bile in a bound form which prevents its reabsorption and promotes its fecal elimination.

*Cesium* is retained more by suckling than by weaned rats (207) and mice (222); the same was found for *plutonium* (19).

The absorption of water-soluble *iron* complexes is high during the first two weeks of life in the rat; thereafter absorption gradually decreases to about 25% at 30 days of age (88).

## Absorption of Vitamins

Only $B_{12}$ absorption was studied during development. It was found that in animals born mature, i.e., guinea pigs, the ability of the small intestine to accumulate $B_{12}$ is fully developed at birth; on the other hand, in rats (born immature) the adult level of ability is attained at the beginning of the fourth week of life. The amount of intrinsic factor in the stomach of rats is low within the first 10 days of life and rises

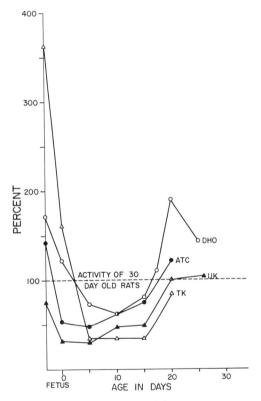

Fig. 11. Activity of dehydroorotase-DHO ($\bigcirc$), aspartate transcarbamylase-ATC ($\bullet$), uridine kinase-UK ($\blacktriangledown$) and thymidine kinase-TK ($\triangledown$) in the small intestines of rats of various ages. Abscissa: age in days. F = fetuses. Ordinate: activities expressed as percentage of activities found in one-month old rats. Constructed from data in (128).

considerably between days 10 and 20 (29). In agreement with this, absorption of cyanocobalamin decreases after weaning as judged by its retention (343). Gallagher (97) concludes that $B_{12}$ absorption in suckling rats occurs by a pinocytic mechanism.

## CHANGES OF ENZYME ACTIVITIES RELATED TO GENERAL METABOLISM OF ENTEROCYTES

For a brief review of data on developmental changes of enzymes in the rat not directly related to digestive and absorptive functions of the

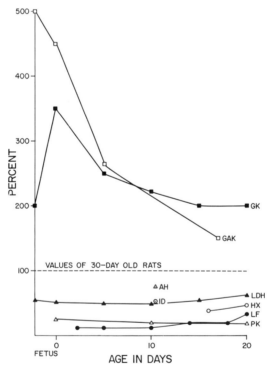

**Fig. 12.** Activity of various enzymes in the small intestines of rats of different ages. Abscissa: age in days, $F$ = fetuses. Ordinate: activity expressed as percentage of activity formed in one-month old rats. ■ = glycerokinase—GK (331). □ = galactokinase—GAK (60). ▽ = aconitate hydratase—AH (25). ⊗ = isocitrate dehydrogenase—ID (25). ▲ = Lacticodehydrogenase—LDH (13). ○ = hexokinase —HX (306). ● = formation of lactate (from glucose)—LF (306). △ = pyruvat-kinase—PK (107).

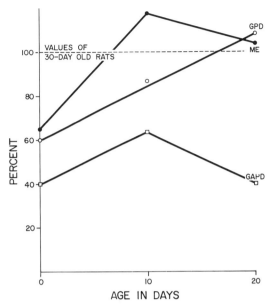

**Fig. 13.** Activity of glycerophosphatedehydrogenase—GPD (○), glycerylaldehyd dehydrogenase—GAPD (□), and malic enzyme—ME (●) in homogenates of small intestine of rats of various ages. Abscissa: age in days. Ordinate: activities expressed as percentage of activities found in one-month old rats. Constructed from data in (107).

small intestine see Figs. 11 to 13. The changes in the enzymes of the *de novo* pathway of pyrimidine biosynthesis (aspartate transcarbamylase and dihydroorotase) and in two enzymes of the salvage pathway (uridine kinase and thymidine kinase) during the ontogeny of the rat are presented in Fig. 11. Their low activity during the suckling period correlates well with the previously determined slow rate of cell renewal in this period in rats (52, 185) and mice (103, 321). Figures 12 and 13 summarize developmental changes in various enzymes of cell metabolism as they were studied in the rat with biochemical methods.

Histochemically it was found that the activities of glucose-6-phosphate dehydrogenase, 6-phosphogluconate dehydrogenase, isocitrate dehydrogenase, succinicdehydrogenase, glutamate dehydrogenase, and monoaminoxidase increase from low in suckling rat to higher in weaned rats. The activities of malate dehydrogenase, α-glycerophosphate dehydrogenase, lactate dehydrogenase, β-hydroxybutyrate dehydrogenase, and NADH diaforase, however, are already high in suckling animals and do not change substantially after weaning (198).

## THE DEVELOPMENT OF REGIONAL DIFFERENCES
## OF THE SMALL AND LARGE INTESTINE

It is known that different parts of the intestinal tube of adult mammals possess different capacities to handle nutrients and other material, thus showing a "specialization" of different sections (32). Studies on developing mammals, including man, have shown that the adult pattern often develops during ontogeny. Data summarized below show that among other things, the comparison of different parts of the small and large intestine during development is important also to an understanding of the changing capacity of functions of the intestine during ontogeny, since concentration of attention on only one section might often be misleading (e.g., changes of activities of lysosomal enzymes if studied only in the jejunum).

Before we discuss the physiological and biochemical changes, we intend to note several striking changes in the general appearance and morphology of the small and large intestine, as related to the changes of jejunoileal gradient and differences between the small and large intestines. (The detailed description of the development of morphology of the gastrointestinal tract is omitted from this review; the interested reader will find more information in other published reviews (170, 171).

In many animals the ileum of some fetuses or infants differ in color from the ileum of adults. Later in development this difference disappears. This fact was first noticed by von Mollendorf (234) in infant mice. Several investigators later noted (e.g., Clark, 50) this difference in rats. In suckling rats the jejunum is white, the ileum yellow. This yellow color sometimes assumes different tones which vary from brownish to greenish. The color is due to the coloration of mucosa. Von Molendorf (234) described the existence of colloid granules in the epithelial cells which have also been observed by Cornell and Padykula (56). Similar color differences of the ileum have been seen in suckling puppies and in rabbits. The ilea of fetal guinea pig, rabbit, and man are differently colored than adult ilea. In man a dark brownish-green appears after the thirteenth week of embryonic life and increases in intensity up to the twenty-fifth week. This coloring is related to the presence in fetuses of meconium, the colored material being obviously deposited in lysosomes (8, 27, 56). Studies on man (8, 27) show that this material gives a positive reaction for phospholipoproteins and lipfuscin.

On the other hand, histological studies show—as far as the presence of villi is concerned—no difference in morphological appearance of the

small and large intestines in earlier phases of ontogeny. Mucosa of the
large intestine is formed in villi in fetuses of rat, rabbit, cat, and man.
These villi disappear in cat and man during fetal life, whereas in rabbit
and rat they disappear postnatally (49, 67, 142, 158, 210, 225, 260, 261).
A high incidence of cells with large vaculoes has been described in
the ileum of suckling animals absorbing intact proteins.

The biochemical and physiological changes that occur in different
parts of the small intestine are summarized in Table 1. Changes in
the large intestinal functions, compared with the same functions in the
small intestine, have already been discussed. We have prepared a few
figures to illustrate the different types of change. Some functions, such
as the activity of nonspecific esterase or the activity of β-glucosidase
(one increasing during development, the other, decreasing) change during postnatal development in a parallel way both in the jejunum and
the ileum of the rat (Fig. 14). Other functions such as the protein/DNA

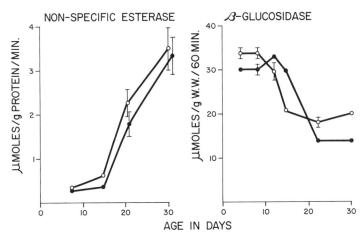

Fig. 14. (a) Activity of nonspecific esterase in the jejunum (○) and ileum (●)
of rats of various ages. Vertical lines denote 2 S.E.M. Abscissa: age in days. Ordinate: /μmoles of substrate split per min per gram of protein (265). (b) β-glucosidase in the jejunum (○) and ileum (●) of rats of various ages. Abscissa: age in
days. Ordinate. μmoles of substrate split per 60 min per g of wet weight. Vertical
lines denote 2 S.E.M. (180).

ratio and RNA/DNA ratio do not differ between jejunum and ileum
during development at all (188). In adult rats a glucose absorption
or phospholipid formation during lipid absorption shows a typical gradient, the activity of these processes being substantially higher in the

**Table 1  Perinatal Development of Regional Differences of the Small Intestine**[a]

| Function | Species | Developmental Stage | Finding | Reference | Note |
|---|---|---|---|---|---|
| **Digestion and Absorption** | | | | | |
| *Carbohydrates* | | | | | |
| Enzymes | | | | | |
| Lactase | Rat | s | $j = i$ | (189) | |
| | Man | f | $j = i$ | (80) | Up to 21 weeks; later activity of jejunum is higher |
| | Dog | s | $j = i$ | (339) | |
| | Cow | n | $j$ fairly as $i$ | (148) | |
| β-Glucosidase | | | | | |
| Sucrase | Rat | s | $j = i$ | (180) | $j =$ also in adults |
| | Man | f | $j = i$ | (157) | Up to 14 weeks; later jejunum has higher activity (see Figure 4). |
| | Man | f | $j$ | (80) | 21 to 38 weeks old |
| | Man | f | $j$ | (64) | 220 mm CR |
| | Dog | s | $j$ fairly as $i$ | (339) | |
| Maltase | Man | f | $j$ | (80) | 21 to 38 weeks old |
| Isomaltase | Man | f | $j$ | (64) | 220 mm CR |
| | Man | f | $j$ | (64) | 220 mm CR |
| | Dog | s | $j$ | (339) | |
| Absorption | | | | | |
| Glucose | Rat | s | $j = i$ | Waitzová, Koldovský (unpublished) | |
| Glucose | Man | f | $j = i$ | (156) | Up to 10 weeks; the older jejunum has higher absorption rate (see Fig. 4). |
| 3-O-methylglucose | | | | | |
| Glucose | Rat | s | $j = i$ | (23) | |
| | Pig | n | $j$ | (271) | |

*Lipids*

| | | | | | |
|---|---|---|---|---|---|
| **Enzymes** | | | | | |
| Lipase | Rat | s | $j = i$ | (278) | Adult, $j = i$ (see Fig. 14). |
| Nonspecific esterase | Rat | s | $j = i$ | (265) | Not known in adults. |
| | Man | f | $i$ | (264) | |
| **Absorption** | | | | | |
| Formation of phospholipids | Rat | s | $j = i$ | (176, 177) | |
| Bile acids absorption | Dog | f | $j$ as $i$ | (297) | |

*Proteins*

| | | | | | |
|---|---|---|---|---|---|
| **Enzymes** | | | | | |
| Protease (substrate casein) | Rat | s | $i$ | (170, p. 102) | Whereas in sucklings the activity of the ileum is six times higher than that of the jejunum, in adults it is only 2.6 times. |
| (substrate nitrocasein) | Rat | s | $i$ | (14) | Same as above |
| | Rat | s | $i$ | (251) | In adults fairly $j = i$. |
| | Man | f | $j = i$ | (133) | In older fetuses ileum activity exceeds that of jejunum (see Fig. 16). |
| Chymotrypsin | Rat | s | $j = i$ | (170, p. 104) | In adult also $j = i$. |
| Trypsin | Rat | s | $i$ | (170) | Absent in adults and suckling starved rats. |
| **Peptidases** | See below | | | | |
| **Absorption** | | | | | |
| Proline | Man | f | $i$ | (208) | In fetuses 14 to 22 weeks old. |
| l-Alanine | Rat | s | | See note (23) | The peak in midileum is less expressed than in adults |

*Miscellaneous*

| | | | | | |
|---|---|---|---|---|---|
| Calcium | Rat | s | $j = i$ | (23) | See Fig. 10 |
| Sulfate | Rat | s | $j = i$ | (22) | See Fig. 10 |
| Vitamin B12 | Rat | s | $i$ | (29) | In adults also ileum activity is higher. |

[a] Enzymes and functions listed here, with the exceptions given in the notes, are found more active in the jejunum than in the ileum of adult mammals.
*Abbreviations used* $f$ = fetus, $n$ = newborn, $s$ = suckling; $j$ means that activity in the jejunum is higher than in the ileum, $i$ = higher activity in the ileum, $j = i$ means that the jejunum and ileum do not differ significantly.

## Table 1 Perinatal Development of Regional Differences of the Small Intestine[a] (Continued)

| Function | Species | Developmental Stage | Finding | Reference | Note |
|---|---|---|---|---|---|
| **Enzymes Related to Other Functions than Above** | | | | | |
| *Acids hydrolases* (lysosomal) *Note.* In adults the activity of the jejunum is usually slightly (10–25%) lower than of the ileum. | | | | | |
| β-Galactosidase | Rat | s | i | (179) | |
| | Rabbit | s | i | (184) | |
| | Guinea pig | s | i | (184) | |
| | Mouse | s | i | (184) | |
| β-Glucuronidase | Rat | s | i | (132) | See Fig. 18. |
| | Rat | s | i | (345) | Histochemically. |
| | Rabbit | s | i | (155) | |
| | Guinea pig | f,n | i | (155) | |
| | Mouse | s | i | (155) | |
| | Pig | s,n | i | (172) | |
| N-Acetyl-β-glucosaminidase | Rat | s | i | (187) | |
| Sulfatase | Rat | s | i | (65, 134, 135) | |
| | Man | f | i | (136) | |
| *Alkaline phosphatase*(s) | | | | | |
| Determination in total homogenates | | | | | |
| Glycerophosphate as substrate | Rat | n | | See note (328) | Appears first in the ileum during development. |
| | Guinea pig | f | i | See note (328) | The same as rat. |
| | Rat | s | i | (251) | |
| | Mouse | s | i | (237) | |
| | Dog | s | j = i | (339) | |
| | Man | f | i | (80) | |
| Phenylphosphate | Mouse | s | i | (237) | |
| | Rat | s | i | (232) | |
| | Mouse | s | j | (2) | Although in adults the activity of the jejunum exceeded that of ileum 30 times, in suckling rats only 1.7 times |
| Naphthylphosphate | Rat | s | i | (65) | |
| | Rat | s | i | (265) | |
| Fraction of homogenates; determination in low speed | Man | f | i | (264) | See Fig. 16b |

| | Species | | | Ref | Notes |
|---|---|---|---|---|---|
| | Rat | s | i | (251) | β-Glyeerophosphate as substrate. |
| | Rat | s | i | (232) | Phenylphosphate as substrate. |
| **Low-speed supernatant** | | | | | |
| | Rat | s | j = i | (251) | |
| | Rat | s | j | (251) | |
| *Peptidases* | | | | | |
| Substrates | | | | | |
| Leucyl-β-naphthylamid | Rat | s | i | (250) | |
| | Man | f | j = i | (133) | In older fetuses the activity of ileum is higher. |
| Glycylglycylglycine | Rat | s | i | (250) | |
| | Man | f | j = i | (133) | Also in older fetuses. |
| Glycylglycine | Rat | s | i | (170) | |
| | Man | f | j = i | (133) | |
| Alanylproline | Rat | s | i | (212) | Also in adults. |
| | Pig | f | j = i | (211) | In older j = i. |
| | Man | f | j = i | (210) | Also in older. |
| Glycyl-leucine | Rat | | Same as alanylproline | | |
| | Pig | | | | |
| | Man | | | | |
| Glycylvaline | Rat | | Same as alanylproline | | |
| | Man | | | | |
| *Encyme of Various Metabolic Pathways* | | | | | |
| Malic enzyme | Rat | s | j | (107) | |
| Pyruvatkinase | Rat | s | j | (107) | |
| Glycerophosphate-dehydrogenase | Rat | s | j | (107) | |
| Glycerylaldehyde-Dehydrogenase | Rat | s | j | (107) | |

*Note.* The following enzymes did not show histochemically substantial differences in activity in enterocytes of the jejunum and ileum of suckling or adult rats: glucose-6-phosphatedehydrogenase, 6-phosphogluconatedehydrogenase, isocitrate-dehydrogenase, succinatedehydrogenase, α-glycerophosphatedehydrogenase, lactatedehydrogenase, β-hydroxy-butyratedehydrogenase, NADH diaphorase [(198)].

a Enzymes and functions listed here, with the exceptions given in the notes, are found more active in the jejunum than in the ileum of adult mammals.

*Abbreviations used* f = fetus, n = newborn, s = suckling; j means that activity in the jejunum is higher than in the ileum, i = higher activity in the ileum, j = i means that the jejunum and ileum do not differ significantly.

jejunum. As shown in Fig. 15, during the suckling period there is no difference between the jejunum and the ileum in their capacity to transport glucose or phospholipids. In human fetuses, also, such a diversion of jejunum and ileum occurs during development. Although glucose

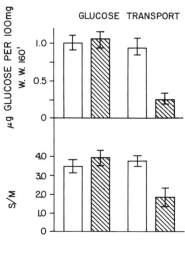

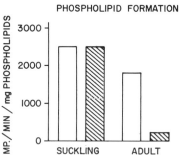

Fig. 15.    (a) Transport of glucose by everted sacs of jejunum ( □ ) and ileum ( ■ ) of suckling (*left pairs*) and adult rats (*right pairs*). Short vertical lines denote 2 S.E.M. Ordinate: (*Upper part*), µg of glucose transferred to serosal fluid per 100 mg wet weight per 60 minutes; (*lower part*) S/M ratio (ratio of final concentration of glucose in the serosal fluid and in the mucosal fluid) (Waitzová and Koldovský, unpublished). (b) Incorporation of $^{32}$P into the phospholipids during in vitro absorption of fat in jejunum and ileum of suckling rats. Arrangement similar to that in (a). Ordinate: imp/min-mg of phospholipids. Constructed from data in (178).

absorption, activity of sucrase (Fig. 4), and activity or protease and alkaline phosphatase (Fig. 16) are the same in 2-month-old fetuses, later the transport capacity for glucose and the activity of sucrase increase in the jejunum. On the other hand, the protease, aminopeptidase, and alkaline phosphatase activities increase in the ileum, thus showing substantially higher activities in the ileum in older fetuses. In the case of alkaline phosphatase this is later reversed (Fig. 16). Figure 10 illustrates a situation in which the functional capacity (transport of calcium and sulfate) does not differ in suckling rats in different parts of the small intestine. Later in development one of the portions (ileum

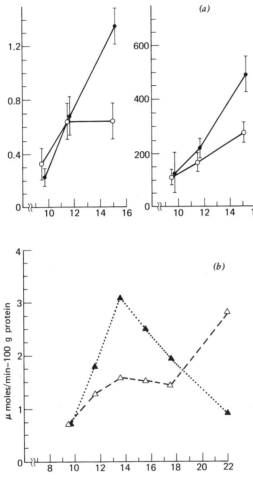

**Fig. 16.** (*a*) Development of proteolytic (*left*) and aminopeptidase (*right*) activities in human fetus small intestine. ○ = jejunum; ● = ileum; short vertical lines = 2 S.E. Abscissa: age of fetuses in weeks (postconceptional). Ordinates: left = $\triangle E^{360}$/g wet weight/60 min; right = $\mu$moles of substrate split/60 min-g wet weight. According to data on (133). Alkaline phosphatase activity in the supernatants of homogenates from the proximal and distal thirds of the small intestine of human fetuses. Abscissa: age in weeks after conception. Ordinate: $\mu$mole of liberated $\beta$-naphthol/min-100 g of protein. Jejunum (△), ileum (▲). Data taken from (264).

or duodenum) becomes the only part of the small intestine in which this function is present.

Figure 17 shows that peptidase splitting leucyl-$\beta$-naphthylamide activity increases in jejunum during development, thus reversing the ratio of activity between the jejunum and the ileum.

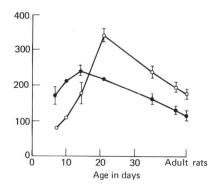

Fig. 17.  Activity of peptidase (substrate leucyl-$\beta$-naphtylamide) in small intestines of rats of various ages. Ordinate: $\Delta E/$ minute-g wet weight of mucosa. Abscissa: age in days. Short vertical lines denote 2 S.E.M. Jejunum (○); ileum (●). Taken from (250).

Acid hydrolases were found to show a striking developmental pattern. Acid $\beta$-galactosidase (179), sulfatase (65, 132, 134, 135), glucosaminidase (187), and $\beta$-glucuronidase (132) decrease slowly after birth in the jejunum of the rat, whereas in the ileum, starting from activities close to those found in the jejunum, they increase to a peak at the end of the suckling period and later decrease again abruptly. This is demonstrated for $\beta$-glucuronidase in Fig. 18. Figure 18 also shows that this phenomenon is not restricted to the rat but can be found in such other species as pig, guinea pig, mouse, and rabbit. In guinea pig the increase in the ileum occurred before birth. A similar transient increase in the ileum was observed for the alkaline phosphatase (found in the 20,000 $\times$ g supernatant) both in human fetuses (Fig. 16) and in postnatal rats (Fig. 19). According to morphological studies, this alkaline phosphatase is also localized in lysosomes (344, 345).

The unusually high activity of lysosomal acid $\beta$-galactosidase, $\beta$-glucuronidase, and N-acetyl-$\beta$-glucosoaminidase in the ileum of suckling rats is also accompanied by a different distribution along the height of the villus. Figure 20 shows that, although neutral $\beta$-galactosidase (true lactase), which served here for comparison, is higher in the upper part of the villus, both in the jejunum and ileum of suckling and adult rats (as other disaccharidases), the acid $\beta$-galactosidase activity decreases along the height of the villus only slightly in adult rats and in the jejunum of suckling rats. In the ileum of suckling rats a steep

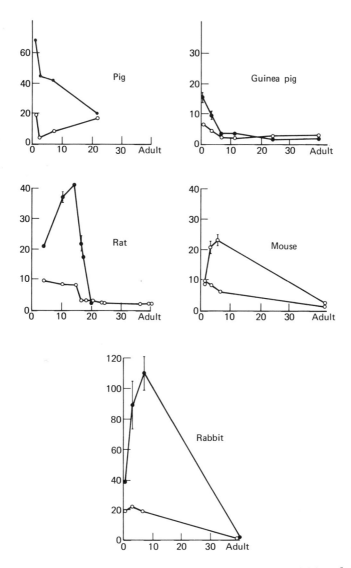

**Fig. 18.** Postnatal changes of β-glucuronidase activity in jejunum (○) and ileum (●) in different mammals. Except in mice, estimations were made with mucosal homogenates; in mice homogenates of the whole intestinal wall were used. Abscissa: age in days. Substrate: phenolphtaleinglucuronide, 0.001 M, pH 4.5. Ordinate: activity given as micrograms of phenolphthalein liberated/60 min-mg of wet wt. Differences described in test are statistically significant at least for $p < 0.01$. Data for pigs (172); rats (132); other animals (155).

gradient (villus to crypts) was found for both mentioned enzymes, a decrease that correlated with the quantity of lysosomes along the height of the villus, as described histologically (101). This decreasing gradient (from tip of the villus toward the crypts) is found in rats for maltase, sucrase, dipeptidase (253), and enterokinase (254), enzymes with digestive functions. This type of distribution contrasts with the distribution pattern of other enzymes. Enzymes related to cell metabolism (e.g.,

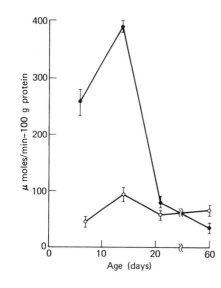

Fig. 19. Development of alkaline phospholase activity in supernatant (22000 g/min–10 min) of jejunum (O) and ileum (●) of rats. Short vertical lines denote 2 S.E.M. Ordinate: μmoles of substrate split/min–100 g protein. Abscissa: age in days (265).

succindehydrogenase) do show no gradient along the height of the villus; enzymes related to pyrimidine and purine metabolism (cell division) show a reverse gradient (i.e., the highest activity is found in the cells) (96, 128). With this in mind, we can speculate about the digestive function of lysosomes in the ileum of suckling rats. These examples, together with the other functions reviewed in Table 1, show that the functional significance of different parts of the small intestine changes during development. The functional significance of high activities of hydrolases in the ileum of suckling animals was often related to the absorption of intact proteins.

Finally, I would like to mention the question of factors that influence the appearance of jujunoileal differences during development. It has been suggested (5) that food coming from the oral end of the tube is responsible for formation of this gradient. This might explain many of the jejunoileal gradients in which peak activities are found in the proximal portions. It is less easy, of course, to use this explanation for

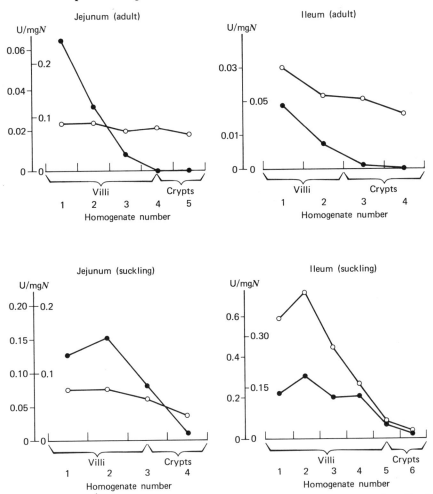

**Fig. 20.** Activity of β-galactosidases in different layers of the intestinal wall of jejunum (*left*) and ileum (*right*) of adult (*upper part*) and suckling (*lower part*) rats. Ordinate: μmoles of substrate split/min–mg of nitrogen. Abscissa gives the portion of sections along the height of the villus. ○ = acid β-galactosidase; ● = neutral β-galactosidase. Adapted from (253).

the development of gradients of functions with their peaks in distal parts of the small intestine. The same argument could be made for the existence of jejunoileal gradients in fetuses, as, for example, the development of jejunoileal gradient of sucrase of glucose transport because the amniotic fluid with substrates for these functions is swallowed in utero. Experiments mentioned below suggest that in the development of jejunoileal gradients hormonal regulation is involved as well. The activity of sucrase is almost entirely absent in the small intestine of suckling rats and can be evoked precociously by the application of cortisone, as we discuss later. In adult rats this enzyme shows a typical distribution along the length of the small intestine, with a decrease toward the distal parts. We have asked ourselves whether cortisone applied in the suckling period will cause differential effects in the jejunum and ileum. Figure 21 shows that cortisone evoked a higher increase in specific activity of sucrase in the jejunum than in the ileum. In other experiments the rate of increase of total sucrase activity in the jejunum and ileum was plotted (290) in order to compare the half-life of the increase. The values of half-life were found to be close in both parts (26 to 27 hours). The experiments thus indicate that the difference between the response of the sucrase activity in the jejunum and that in the ileum cannot be accounted as the result of different rates of increase but is a result of different amounts of sucrase-forming units ("reactive sites"). Correlation with the amount of microvilli in different parts of the small intestine is possible. These experiments, when compared with previously mentioned data, suggest that both food intake and endocrine regulation may be factors responsible for the development of a discrete distributional pattern for various functions along the length of the small intestine.

### Changes in Colon

As previously noted, during earlier stages of development of the human fetus the large intestine histologically resembles the small intestine.

Masnerová, Kaldovsky, and Kubát (219), in agreement with other authors, have shown that in adult rats no detectable alkaline phosphatase activity is present in the enterocytes of the large intestine. On the contrary, this activity is positive during the first weeks of postnatal life of the rat and it disappears after the twentieth day. At the same time, as activity decreases in the enterocytes, there is a rise in the endothelium. It has been speculated that the large intestine might thus also possess some transport mechanisms present only in the small intestine of adult animals. Actually, it has been found that the large intestine of newborn and suckling rats actively transports sulfate (22), calcium, and 3-o-methylglucose (23) (Fig. 10). These active transport capacities diminish as the weaning period approaches (as the alkaline phosphatase does also) and are nearly absent in 5-week-old rats.

In the earlier phases of human fetal development the large intestine possesses activity of sucrase and several dipeptidases. *Sucrase* was found in the large intestine of human fetuses (C—R length 6.5 to 20.0 cm) (64). Comparison of the developmental changes in the large intestine and small intestine shows that in 10-week-old fetuses the activity of both intestines is the same; the large intestine activity does not change, whereas the activity in the small intestine substantially increases (157) (Fig. 4). Several *dipeptidases* (substrates: alanyl-glutamic acid, alanyl-proline, glycyl-glycine, glycyl-leucine, and glycyl-valine) were shown by Lindberg (210) to be present in the large intestine of human fetuses (C—R length 6.5 to 20.0 cm) in the same activity as in the small intestine. No comparison was made with activity in adult subjects. In adult rats it is known that these activities are lower in the large than in  the small intestine (160).

Finally, several enzymes, more related to the metabolism of the cell, were compared in their activity in the small and large intestine during development. Although specific activity changes in most of them during postnatal development in the rat, the ratio between their activity in the small and large intestines does not change substantially. This was proved histochemically by Kubát and Koldovský (198) for glucose-6-phosphate dehydrogenase, 6-phosphogluconate dehydrogenase, isocitrate dehydrogenase, α-glycerophosphate dehydrogenase, glutamate dehydrogenase, β-hydroxybutyrate dehydrogenase, malate dehydrogenase, lactate dehydrogenase, monoamine oxidase, succinate dehydrogenase, NADH diaphorase, and biochemically by Hahn and Skala (107) for α-glycerophosphate dehydrogenase, pyruvate kinase, glyceraldehyde dehydrogenase, and malic enzyme. Although general metabolism of the large intestinal enterocytes does not differ with age from that of the small intestinal entercytes, in some specific functions related mainly to transport the large intestine during postnatal development actually "loses" the functions that during adult life "belong" only to the small intestine. The reasons for the existence and for the disappearance of these functions are unknown.


## THE FACTORS INFLUENCING THE NORMAL DEVELOPMENT OF GASTROINTESTINAL FUNCTIONS

Almost simultaneously with the effort to define differences in functional equipment of the gastrointestinal tract during different developmental periods, the question of factors responsible for the differences and development from one stage to another has attracted the attention of investigators. As in the development of other mammalian systems, the effects both of endocrines and dietary changes were studied. We discuss first the effect of hormones. These experiments have more compact information than those based on the effect of diet. We point out the possibility that change of diet (including starvation) or just the handling of an animal may function as a stress, and the effects noted in these experiments in suckling animals might be at least partly the results of stimulation of the adrenals.

## Effects of Hormones

The object of most studies was to elucidate the role of steroids; we discuss this subject first.

### Maturative Effect of Adrenal Steroids

Most of the studies were performed on mice and rats; other animals were used rarely. Findings are presented here from three aspects. First we summarize the functions that are influenced by adrenal steroids during the suckling period. Then we discuss the sensitivity of reactive systems as it depends on the type of steroid, the dose of steroid, and postnatal age. Finally we review experiments in which the dynamics of cortisone-evoked changes were studied (i.e., in which an attempt was made to show how fast the cortisone reaction is and how the cortisone-evoked reactions correlate with the cell migration along the villus and in which the villus changes are detected first).

*The effects of various adrenal steroids on the functions* of the developing gastrointestinal tract are summarized in Table 2.

## Different Sensitivities of Maturing Systems of the Small Intestine

### Comparison of Different Steroids

The effect of steroids was compared on the development of two functions, namely, increase of alkaline phosphatase (240) in duodenum of mice and cessation of absorption of antibodies in rats (112). In experiments of Moog and Thomas (240) the effect of cortisone acetate was highest; the effect of hydrocortisone acetate was close to cortisone; corticosterone and 11-dehydrocortisone were less effective. Progesterone and DOCA were effective only in doses six times higher than the drugs previously mentioned. Hydrocortisone as free alcohol and tetrahydrocortisone were almost without effect. Estradiol benzoate and testosterone propionate were ineffective in 9-day-old mice, whereas in 14-day-old males testosterone exerted a strong effect. In Halliday's experiment (112) both DOCA and cortisone acetate decreased the absorption of antibodies in suckling rats; aldosterone, progesterone, testosterone, and stilbestrol were without effect.

### Changes of Sensitivity to Cortisone with Age and Dependence on Dose

All described effects of cortisone are peculiar to the suckling period. Cortisone is usually without effect in weaned animals. Further, it was found that during the suckling period the sensitivity to cortisone changes. We have already mentioned in Table 2 that short-term (four days) cortisone application is without effect on cell migration, whereas long-term application (eight days) has an effect (129). Moog and Thomas (240) have shown that the same dose of cortisone evokes a higher response in 14-day-old than in 9-day-old mice, having no effect on 2-day-old mice. Clark (50) has observed that the application of cortisone "matures" enterocytes in 8-day-old animals regularly, whereas the effect on 5-day-old animals is irregular. These experiments indicate that at the beginning of the suckling period the response to cortisone is lower and that the systems respond more when the period of their normally occurring change (usually weaning) nears. We have tested this in rats, studying the effect of cortisone on sucrase (an enzyme that increases) and on acid $\beta$-galactosidase (an enzyme that decreases during the weaning period). Data from these experiments are summarized in Figs. 21 and 22. The results give one common conclusion: the reactivity of both enzymes increases with age; maximal effect is seen closest to weaning. The reactions of these two enzymes differ, however. Sucrase is induced in the youngest animals used. Acid-$\beta$-galactosidase does not respond in 8-day-old animals; its decrease could be evoked only in the middle of the suckling period. The highest dose used (5 mg/100 g b.w.) has almost the same effect on the sucrase in all age groups studied. The change of sensitivity with age could be detected only with the low doses. In the case of acid-$\beta$-galactosidase all doses used showed an increase of sensitivity with age. Finally, the dose dependency could be shown with the sucrase both in the jejunum and in the ileum, whereas in the acid-$\beta$-galactosidase it could be shown only in preparations from ileum.

### The Dynamics of Cortisone-Evoked Changes

An important aspect of cortisone-evoked changes is the rate of the reaction. In other words, when can we expect to detect the changes evoked by cortisone? The enterocytes migrate along the height of the villi of the small intestinal mucosa more slowly in suckling rats than in adult ones. It takes 96 hours after injection of thymidine for labeled cells to appear in suckling rats at the top of the villus (129, 184). The

**Table 2  Effect of Adrenal Steroids on Gastrointestinal Functions in Suckling Animals[a]**

| Function | Animal | Steroid | Response | Note | Reference |
|---|---|---|---|---|---|
| Pancreas: | | | | | |
| Weight | Rat | Cortisone | Increase | * | (291) |
| RNA/DNA | Rat | Cortisone | Increase | * | (291) |
| Lipase | Rat | Cortisone | Increase | | (278) |
| | Rat | Cortisone | | * | (291) |
| Amylase | Rat | Corticosterone | Increase | | (274) |
| Protease (Trypsin) | Rat | Cortisone | Increase | * | (291) |
| Small intestine: | | | | | |
| *Morphology* | | | | | |
| Weight of the jejunum | Rat | Cortisone | Increase | | Own unpublished results |
| Weight of the ileum | Rat | Cortisone | No change or decrease no change | | Own unpublished results |
| Protein/DNA | Rat | Cortisone | | | (188) |
| RNA/DNA | Rat | Cortisone | Increase | | (188) |
| Depth of crypts, mitotic index, rate of cell migration | Rat | Hydrocortisone | Increase | This effect was seen only after eight days of application; shorter application was without effect. | (129) |
| Appearance of entero-cytes (i.e., presence of vacuoli, inclusions, and development of Golgi apparatus) | Rat | Cortisone | "Matures" | | (50) |
| | Mouse | Cortisone | "Matures" | | (256) |

| | | | | | |
|---|---|---|---|---|---|
| Lengthening of the microvilli | Mouse | Cortisone | Increase | | (256) |
| Number of Goblet cells | Mouse | Cortisone | Increase | | (50) |
| *enzyme activities* | | | | | |
| Alkaline phosphatase | Rat embryo | Cortisone | Increase | Applied to mother | (280) |
| | Rat embryo | Cortisone | Increase | Applied to embryo | (327) |
| | Rat embryo | Adrenalectomy of the mother | Increase | | (330) |
| | Mouse | Cortisone | Increase | Effect in duodenum, not in jejunum; changes also in substrates affinity | (237) |
| | Mouse | Cortisone | Increase | Effect in duodenum only; also comparison with other steroids | (235, 240) |
| Sucrase | Mouse | Adrenalectomy prevents increase | | | (236) |
| | Rat | Hydrocortisone | Increase | The same effect found in tissue cultures | (75) |
| | Rat | Adrenalectomy, corticosterone | Delay in increase restores the normal increase | | (180) |
| Neutral β-galactosidase (lactase) | Rat | Adrenalectomy | Delay in decrease | | Own unpublished results |
| Acid β-galactosidase | Rat | Adrenalectomy | Slows the decrease | | (179) |
| | Rat | Corticosterone normalizes the effect of adrenalectomy | | | (181) |
| | Rat | Cortisone | Decrease | | (189) |

**Table 2  Effect of Adrenal Steroids on Gastrointestinal Functions in Suckling Animals (*Continued*)**

| Function | Animal | Steroid | Response | Note | Reference |
|---|---|---|---|---|---|
| β-Glucuronidase | Rat | Adrenalectomy | Slows the decrease | | (132) |
| | Rat | Cortisone | Decrease | | Own unpublished results |
| N-Acetyl-β-glucos-aminidase | Rat | Cortisone | Decrease | | Own unpublished results |
| Arylsulphatase | Rat | Adrenalectomy | Slows the decrease | | (135) |
| Nonspecific esterase | Rat | Adrenalectomy | Inhibits the increase | | (265) |
| | Rat | Cortisone to adrenalectomized rats normalizes the increase | | | (265) |
| *Other Functions* | | | | | |
| Absorption of antibodies | Rat | Cortisone | Decrease | | (50) |
| | | | | | (112) |
| Absorption of B12 | Pig | Cortisone | Decrease | | (262) |
| | Rat | Cortisone | Abolished | | (97) |
| Absorption of Cu | Rat | Cortisone | Reduces absorption; increases secretion into the bile | | (233) |

[a] Same treatment was found to be without effect on adults, except when no comparison was done. These experiments are then denoted by *.

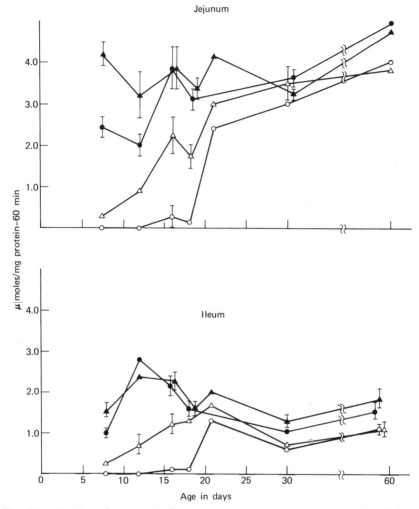

**Fig. 21.** Activity of sucrase in homogenates of jejunum (*upper part*) and ileum (*lower part*) of rats of various ages. Ordinate: μmoles of substrate split/mg of protein = 60 min. Abscissa: age in days. Short vertical lines denote 2 S.E.M. ◯ = intact rats, △ = rats injected daily for four days with 0.5 mg of cortisone/100 g b.w. = 24 hr, ● = rats injected daily for four days with 2.0 mg of cortisone/100 g b.w. = 24 hr, ▲ = rats injected daily for four days with 5 mg of cortisone/100 g b.w. = 24 hr. (130).

185

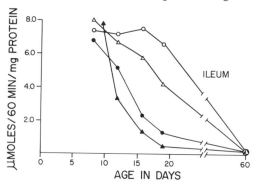

Fig. 22.    Activity of acid β-galactosidase in homogenates of ileum of rats of various ages. Same arrangement of symbols as in Fig. 21. Data constructed from (189).

migration from the crypt-villus junction lasts 72 hours, as has been found also by Clarke and Hardy (52). The application of cortisone in a dose of 5 mg/per 100 g b.w. for 4 days does not change this rate of migration, as has been found repeatedly (129, 130).

Mature cells appear for the first time in normal rats between day 18 and day 21 at the bottom of the villus. The cells on the upper part of the villus still look immature. Such a picture is seen in 10-day-old rats injected with cortisone 48 hours before (50). Doell, Rosen, and Kretchmer (76) have shown that 24 hours after cortisone injection the first detectable sucrase protein (using fluorescent antibodies) is found near the base of the villus only and that 48 hours later fluorescence has extended more distally along the villi. Herbst and Koldovský in unpublished experiments have compared direct determination of sucrase activity in sections taken from different heights of the villus and simultaneously determined the rate of cell migration. (Cortisone and thymidine were injected into animals at the same time.) Data presented in Fig. 23 confirm the observations of Doell et al. (76) and prove that the appearance of sucrase is related to newly appearing cells. As the cells migrate, more sucrase activity is present along the height of the villus. In addition, the sucrase activity of the homogenate increases. Figure 23 shows that the increase of sucrase after the administration of cortisone could be detected first in homogenates of the total wall of the jejunum 24 hours later. This agrees with data previously published by Doell and Kretchmer (74). A significant increase is seen after 48 hours. This two-day period to detect changes caused by cortisone was described also for the increase of alkaline phosphatase in the duodenum (240), cessation of absorption of antibodies (112), and changes in morphological appearance (50). Experiments now under way in our

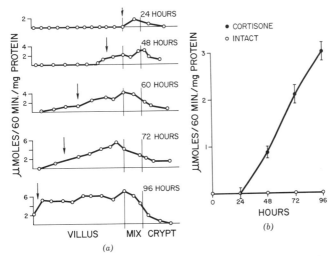

**Fig. 23.** Changes in activity of sucrase in homogenates of different layers of the jejunal wall (*a*) and of the entire jejunal wall (*b*) of 9-day old rats at different periods after daily injections of cortisone—5 mg/100 g b.w. = 24 hr. (*b*) Short vertical lines denote 2 S.E.M.; ● = rats injected with cortisone, ○ = intact littermates (130).

laboratory show that in a cortisone-evoked decrease of acid-$\beta$-galactosidase and other lysomal enzymes ($\beta$-glucuronidase, $N$-acetyl-OMH-glucosaminidase) a different "time schedule" may exist. This also may explain why Danovitch and Laster (65) saw no effect of cortisone on arylsulphatase activity, since they looked for the effect 24 and 48 hours after injection.

## Effect of Other Hormones

Not many experiments can be found in the literature. Removal of *epiphysis* in the rat fetus changes the morphological development of the ileum (257). *Thymectomy* in newborn hamsters disturbs the regular appearance of crypts in weaned animals (114). We have mentioned the effects of progesterone and stilbestrol. Injection of *thyroxin* into suckling rats increases pancreatic weight, RNA/DNA ration, and amylase activity (291).

### Experiments Testing the Effect of Dietary Changes on Various Functions

As we noted in the introduction, the type of diet consumed by animals changes substantially during weaning, and, as we have seen, most functional changes occur during weaning. Various experiments have thus been designed to determine the effect of food changes on the normal developmental pattern of different functions.

The length and shape of villi change in the rat at the time of weaning. Verzar and McDougall (332) fed weaned rats a milk diet for five months, but the shape of the villi was the same as in normally fed animals. Brodskij (43) attempted unsuccessfully to influence by diet the presence of vacuoles in ileal enterocytes of suckling rats.

Only artificial feeding of rats 9 to 15 days old is known to influence the morphological appearance of the intestine. Herbst and Sunshine (129) found under such conditions an increase of relative intestinal weight, mitotic index, and depth of jejunal crypt columns.

Lactase increases before birth in rats and rabbits. Doell and Kretchmer (74) have correlated this increase with the rise of lactose in the blood of the mother, which also occurs• during the last few days of gestation. Surgical removal of the mammary glands of pregnant rabbits did not, however, prevent the rise in lactase activity.

Reports about the effect of variation of lactose intake during the weaning period are contradictory. Although Weinland (337) and Plimmer (272) found a delay in the decrease of lactase as a result of feeding a high-lactose diet, Heilskov (122) found no effect. Also, intraperitoneal application of lactose did not prevent the decrease of lactase in infant rats (74).

Whereas additional feeding of sucrose and isomaltose did not increase (induce) the activity of sucrase and isomaltase in suckling rats (282), artificial feeding of rats 9 to 15 days old induced the sucrase precociously (129). Weaning of rats in the presence of the mother on a low-carbohydrate diet resulted in a lower rate of absorption of glucose in 20- to 30-day-old rats (90) and in rats 2 to 3 months old (100). Herschel, Hill, and Porter (137) were unable to show that *pepsin* activity was initiated precociously by feeding roughage to very young calves.

Activity of alkaline phosphatase in the duodenum of suckling mice is increased by starvation, by precocious feeding of a solid diet, and by feeding cows' milk (235). Moog mentions the probable accompanying effect of the new dietary treatment (i.e., the effect of stress). Prolongation of suckling in younger suckling mice by replacing the original mother with a foster mother does not prevent the usual increase of alkaline phosphatase (235). This almost excludes the existence of a factor present in milk at the end of the lactation period which could stimulate the increase. Similarly designed studies were performed in rats to influence the absorption of antibodies by changing the diet. Halliday (110) has found that suckling rats fostered on the mother of litters older than themselves continued to absorb antibodies beyond the age at which the foster mother's own young would have ceased to do so. Young rats fostered on the mothers of litters younger than themselves ceased to absorb antibodies at the normal age, although the foster mother's own young would have continued to do so. Young rats prevented from taking solid food and compelled to live entirely on milk beyond the normal age nevertheless ceased to absorb antibodies at 20 days of age. Although change in the milk regimen did not influence the length of the period of absorption of intact protein, in another experiment Halliday (112) showed that removing 16-day-old rats from their mother and feeding them for two days on glucose and water caused a precocious cessation of antibody absorption. The last-mentioned finding, however, might not be the effect of early dietary change but rather an effect of stress—a corticoid effect. A different situation was found in other mammals. In the pig absorption of antibodies and large molecules ceases 24 to 36 hours after birth. It was found also that starving these animals (i.e., preventing food intake) extends this absorption period up to 86 to 106 hours (203, 262). Piglets deprived of colostrum and fed a glucose diet only are able to absorb gammaglobulin at 2 weeks of age (215). Lecce and Morgan (203) have further shown that early feeding shortens the period during which proteins can be transferred in piglets. The effect of milk intake is direct because pigs with ligated small intestines did cease absorption of antibodies anterior to the ligature but absorbed antibodies in the posterior segment (262, 263).

Lecce et al. (202) analyzed this mechanism of "closure." They first found that the time during which polyvinylpyrrolidone can be absorbed is longer in piglets that had started to consume colostrum from the mother animal than in those given cow colostrum. They further showed (203) that the more cow colostrum consumed by the piglet, the less polyvinylpyrrolidone was absorbed.

"Closure" is caused by defatted, deproteinized fractions of cow colostrum or a dialysate of the same colostrum (204). "Closure" also occurs after glucose, lactose, xylose, galactose, and sucrose administration (200).

The effect of the amount of substances consumed is considerable (200, 203). The concentration of the glucose solution, on the other hand, is not decisive.

The sensitivity of the gut to "closure" by glucose develops postnatally, since up to the twelfth postnatal hour glucose was usually without effect (200). If there is "closure," the intestine cannot again be "opened" by further starvation (202). This indicates that a more permanent change occurred and not that some holes are being "filled in." The susceptibility of the gut to "closure" factors is not a function of physiological age at birth because piglets born after a gestation period of four days longer than normal also behave in this way after starvation or feeding (262, 263).

## ACKNOWLEDGMENT

Work on this chapter was supported in part by a grant (AMHD 14531) from the National Institutes of Health, Bethesda, Maryland.
I wish to express my gratitude to authors and publishers for permission to use the following figures: Figs. 3 and 23, *Biochem. J.;* Fig. 5, *Biochim. Biophys. Acta;* Fig. 6, *Arch. Dis. Child.;* Figs. 7a and 8, *J. Physiol. (London);* Fig. 7b, *J. Cell. Biol.;* Fig. 20, *J. Histochem. Cytochem.;* and Figs. 2, 4, 14, and 16–19, S. Karger AG, Basel. Specific references are found in legends to these figures.

## REFERENCES

1. F. Aherne, V. W. Hays, R. C. Evan, and V. C. Speer, *J. Amin. Sci.* **29:** 444 (1969).
2. W. Albrecht, Z. *Kinderheilkunde* **79:** 264 (1957).
3. V. Allfrey, M. Stern, and A. E. Mirsky, *Nature* **169:** 128 (1952).
4. D. H. Alpers, *J. Biol. Chem.* **244:** 1238 (1969).
5. G. G. Altmann and C. P. Leblond, *Amer. J. Anat.* **127:** 15 (1970).
6. M. D. Ames, *AMA J. Dis. Child.* **100:** 252 (1960).
7. D. M. Andersen, *Amer. J. Dis. Child.* **63:** 643 (1942).
8. H. Andersen, F. Bierring, E. N. Mattheiss, J. Egeberg, and F. Bro-Rasmussen, *Acta Path. Microbiol. Scand.* **61:** 377 (1964).
9. N. G. Asp, A. Dahlqvist, and O. Koldovsky, *Gastroenterology* **58:** 591 (1970).
10. J. M. Asplund, R. M. Grummer, and R. Phillips, *J. Anim. Sci.* **21:** 412 (1962).
11. S. Auricchio, A. Rubino, and G. Mürset, *Pediat.* **35:** 944 (1965).
12. S. Auricchio, D. D. Pietra, and A. Vegnente, *Pediat.* **39:** 853 (1967).
13. J. M. Bailey, P. H. Fishman, and P. G. Pentchev, *J. Biol. Chem.* **245:** 559 (1970).
14. K. Baintner and B. Veress, *Experientia,* **26:** 54 (1970).
15. S. J. Baker, V. I. Mathan, and V. Cher, *Lancet,* **ii:** 860 (1963).
16. I. R. Balconi and J. G. Lecce, *Fed. Proc.* **20:** 1357 (1965).
17. W. E. Balfour and R. S. Comline, *J. Physiol.* **148:** 77P (1959).
18. W. E. Balfour and R. S. Comline, *J. Physiol.* **160:** 234 (1962).
19. J. E. Ballou, *Proc. Soc. Exptl. Biol.* **98:** 726 (1958).
20. D. R. Bamford, *Proc. Roy. Soc. (London)* **B166:** 30 (1966).
21. D. R. Bangham, K. R. Hobbs, and R. J. Terry, *Lancet* **ii:** 351, 1958.
22. E. R. Batt, *Amer. J. Physiol.* **217:** 1101 (1969).

23. E. R. Batt and D. Schachter, *Amer. J. Physiol.* **216**: 1064 (1969).

24. R. E. Becker, W. F. Windle, E. E. Barth, and M. D. Schultz, *Surg. Gynecol. Olsted.* **70**: 603 (1940).

25. V. Behnke, H. A. Ketz, and K. Täufel, *Acta. Biol. Med. German* **16**: 514 (1966).

26. R. Berfenstam, R. Jagenburg, and O. Mellander, *Acta Paediat. (Uppsala)* **44**: 348 (1955).

27. F. Bierring, H. Andersen, J. Egeberg, M. Mattheesen, and F. Bro-Rasmussen, *Acta Path. Microbiol. Scand.* **61**: 1365 (1964).

28. E. Blum, A. I. Yarmoschewitsch, and A. I. Yakorotschuk, *Bull. Biol. Med. Exptl. USSR* **11**: 113 (1936).

29. A. Boass and T. H. Wilson, *Amer. J. Physiol.* **204**: 101 (1963).

30. S. W. Boellner, A. G. Beard, and T. C. Panos, *Pediat.* **361**: 542 (1965).

31. A. M. Bongiovanni, *J. Clin. Endocr.* **25**: 658 (1965).

32. G. C. Booth, Effect of Location Along the Small Intestine on Absorption of Nutrients, in *Handb. Physiol., Alimentary Canal,* Amer. Physiol. Soc. section G., **III**: 1513, (1968).

33. L. O. Boréus, *Biol. Neonat.* **11**: 328 (1967).

34. L. O. Boréus, *Acta Physiol. Scand.* **72**: 194 (1968).

35. B. Borgström, B. Lindqvist, and G. Lund, *Amer. J. Dis. Child.* **99**: 338 (1960).

36. F. W. R. Brambell, *Biol. Rev.* **33**: 488 (1958).

37. F. W. R. Brambell, The Transition of Passive Immunity from Mother to Young. Amsterdam-New York: North Holland-American Elsevier, 1970.

38. F. W. R. Brambell, W. A. Hemmings, M. Henderson, M. J. Parry, and W. T. Rowlands, *Proc. Roy. Soc. (London)* **B1361**: 131 (1949).

39. F. W. R. Brambell, R. Halliday, *Proc. Roy. Soc. (London)* **B145**: 170 (1956).

40. F. W. R. Brambell, W. A. Hemmings, M. Henderson, C. L. Oakley, and W. T. Rowlands, *Proc. Roy. Soc. (London)* **B138**: 195 (1951).

41. F. W. R. Brambell, R. Halliday, and I. G. Morris, *Proc. Roy. Soc. (London)* **B149**: 131 (1958).

42. F. W. R. Brambell, R. Halliday, and W. A. Hemmings, *Proc. Roy. Soc. (London),* **B153**: 477 (1961).

43. R. A. Brodskij, *Arch. Anal. Histol. Embryol. USSR* **35**: 64 (1958).

44. P. Brown, M. W. Smith, and R. Witty, *J. Physiol.* **198**: 365 (1968).

45. J. H. Butt and T. H. Wilson, *Amer. J. Physiol.* **215**: 1468 (1968).

46. A. Calingaert and A. Zorzoli, *J. Geront.* **20**: 211 (1965).

47. K. Čapek and J. Jelínek, *Physiol. Bohemoslov* **5**: 76 (1956).

48. E. J. Castle, *Brit. J. Nutr.* **10**: 115 (1956).

49. D. Cho, *Jap. J. Obstet. Gynec.* **14**: 324 (1931).

50. S. L. Clark, *J. Bioph. Bioch. Cytol.* **5**: 41 (1959).

51. R. M. Clarke and R. N. Hardy, *J. Physiol.* **204**: 113 (1969).

52. R. M. Clarke and R. N. Hardy, *J. Physiol.* **204**: 127 (1969).

53. M. I. Cohen, L. M. Gartner, O. O. Blumenfeld, and I. M. Arias, *Pediat. Res.* **3**: 5 (1969).

54. R. S. Comline, H. F. Roberts, and D. A. Titschen, *Nature* **167**: 561 (1951).

55. R. S. Comline, H. F. Roberts, and D. A. Titschen, *Nature* **168**: 84 (1951).

56. R. Cornell and H. A. Padykula, *Anat. Rec.* **151**: 339 (1965).

57. R. Cornell and H. A. Padykula, *Amer. J. Anat.* **125**: 291 (1969).

58. R. K. Crane, *Gastroenterology* **50**: 254 (1966).

59. R. K. Crane, *Ann. Rev. Med.* **19**: 57 (1968).

60. P. Cuatrecases and S. Segal, *J. Biol. Chem.* **240**: 2382 (1965).

61. H. M. Cunningham and G. J. Brisson, *Canad. J. Agr. Sci.* **35**: 371 (1955).

62. H. M. Cunningham and W. M. F. Leat, *Canad. J. Biochem.* **47**: 1013 (1969).

63. R. D. Cutler, *J. Pediat.* **12**: 1 (1938).

64. A. Dahlqvist and T. Lindberg, *Clin. Sci.* **30**: 517 (1966).

65. S. H. Danovitch and L. Laster, *Biochem. J.* **114**: 343 (1969).

66. M. E. Davis and E. L. Potter, *J. Amer. Med. Assoc.* **131**: 1194 (1946).

67. L. V. Davletova, *Zh. Obshch. Biol. USSR* **22**: 201 (1961).

68. H. De Groot and P. Hoogendoom, *Netherland Milk and Dairy J.* **11**: 290 (1957).

69. J. J. Deren, Development of Intestinal Structure and Function, in *Handb. Physiol.* Alimentary Canal, *Amer. Physiol. Soc.*, Section 6, **III**: 1099 (1968).

70. J. J. Deren, Development of Structure and Function in the Fetal and Newborn Stomach, *Amer. J. Clin. Nutr.* **23**: 67 (1970).

71. J. J. Deren, E. W. Strauss, and T. H. Wilson, *Develop. Biol.* **12**: 467 (1965).

72. H. J. Deuel, L. Hallman, and A. Leonard, *J. Nutr.* **20**: 215 (1940).

73. M. Dobiášová, P. Hahn, O. Koldovský, *Biochim. Biophys. Acta 84*, 538 (1969).

74. R. G. Doell, and N. Kretchmer, *Biochim. Biophys. Acta* **62**: 353 (1962).

75. R. G. Doell and N. Kretchmer, *Science* **143**: 42 (1964).

76. R. G. Doell, G. Rosen, and N. Kretchmer, *Proc. Natl. Acad. Sci.* (USA) **54**: 1268 (1965).

77. W. Droese and H. Stolley, *Fette-Seifen-Anstrichmittel-Ernährungsindustrie*, **62**: 281 (1960).

78. V. Dudin, *cit. Salenius* (1962).

79. D. W. Ebers, D. I. Smith, and G. E. Gibbs, *Pediat.* **18**: 800 (1956).

80. E. Eggermont, *Biol. Neonat.* **10**: 266 (1966).

81. K. Ehrhardt, *Munch. Med. Wschr.* **86**: 915 (1939).

82. M. M. El-Nageh, *Am. Med. Vet.* **6**: 3 (1967).

83. M. M. El-Nageh, *Am. Med. Vet.* **6**: 380 (1967).

84. M. M. El-Nageh, *Am. Med. Vet.* **6**: 384 (1967).

85. M. M. El-Nageh, *Am. Med. Vet.* **6**: 400 (1967).

86. M. M. El-Nageh, *Amer. Med. Vet.* **8**: 699 (1968).

87. J. Encrantz and J. Sjövall, *Clin. Chim. Acta* **4**: 793 (1959).

88. E. Ezekiel, *J. Lab. Clin. Med.* **70**: 138 (1967).

89. G. Falk, *Amer. J. Physiol.* **181**: 157 (1955).

90. E. Faltová, P. Hahn, and O. Koldovský, *Proc 5th Nat. Congr. Czech. Physiol. Soc.* 1961, Publ. House Chechoslov. Med. Sci., Prague.

91. E. Faltová, P. Hahn, and O. Koldovský, *Fiziol. Zh. USSR* **48**: 1392 (1962); Engl. Trans. *Fed. Proc.* **22**: T941, 1963.

92. S. Farber, C. L. Moddoch, and H. Schwachmann, cited in Smith (298).

93. M. S. Feinsteine and C. A. Smith, *Pediat.* **7**: 19 (1951).

94. J. D. Fletcher and E. T. Waters, *Biochem. J.* **31**: 1830 (1937).

95. L. S. Fomina, *Vop. Med. Chim.* **6**: 176 (1960).

96. R. Fortin-Magana, R. Hurwitz, J. J. Herbst, N. Kretchmer, Science **167**: 1627 (1970).

97. N. D. Gallagher, *Nature* **222**: 877 (1969).

98. C. Garbarsch, *Histochemie* **18**: 168 (1969).

99. C. Garbarsh and F. A. v. Bulow, *Histochemie* **20**: 201 (1969).

100. J. M. Ginsburg, and F. W. Heggeness, *J. Nutr.* **96**: 494 (1969).

101. D. O. Graney, *J. Anat.* **123**: 227 (1968).

102. J. H. Graves, *J. Immunol.* **91**: 251 (1963).

103. R. D. Grey, *Develop. Biol.* **18**: 501 (1968).

104. C. Griswold and A. T. Shohl, *Amer. J. Dis. Child.* **30**: 541 (1925).

105. R. Gschwind, *Amer. Pediat.* **175**: 169 (1950).

106. B. Hadorn, G. Zoppi, H. Shmerling, A. Prader, I. McIntyre, and C. M. Anderson, *J. Pediat.* **73**: 39 (1968).

107. P. Hahn aňd J. Skala, *Biol. Neonate,* **18**: 433 (1971).

108. P. Hahn, and O. Koldovský, *Utilization of Nutrients During Postnatal Development.* Oxford: Pergamon, 1967.

109. R. Halliday, *Proc. Roy. Soc. (London)* **B143**: 408 (1955).

110. R. Halliday, *Proc. Roy. Soc. (London)* **B145**: 179 (1956).

111. R. Halliday, *Proc. Roy. Soc. (London)* **B148**: 92 (1957).

112. R. Halliday, *J. Endocrin.* **18**: 56 (1959).

113. R. Halliday, and R. A. Keckwick, *Proc. Roy. Soc. (London)* **B153**: 541 (1960).

114. R. C. Hard, N. Martinez, and N. Good, *Nature* **204**: 455 (1969).

115. R. N. Hardy, *J. Physiol.* **204**: 607 (1969).

116. R. N. Hardy, *J. Physiol.* **204**: 633 (1969).

117. R. N. Hardy, *J. Physiol.* **205**: 435 (1969).

118. R. N. Hardy, *J. Physiol.* **205**: 453 (1969).

119. J. T. Harries, and A. J. Fraser, *Biol. Neonat.* **12**: 186 (1968).

120. P. A. Hartman, V. W. Hays, R. O. Baker, L. W. Neagl, and D. V. Catron, *J. Anim. Sci.* **20**: 114 (1961).

121. S. Hebert and A. Demay, *C. R. Soc. Biol.* **150**: 335 (1956).

122. N. S. Heilskov, *Acta Physiol. Scand.* **24**: 86 (1951).

123. N. D. Heizer, and L. Laster, *Biochim. Biophys. Acta* **185**: 409 (1969).

124. H. F. Helander, *Gastroenterology* **56**: 35 (1969).

125. H. F. Helander, *Gastroenterology* **56**: 53 (1969).

126. H. Heller, *J. Physiol.* **106**: 245 (1947).

127. J. Heller, *Physiol. Bohemoslov.* **12**: 526 (1963).

128. J. J. Herbst, R. Fortin-Magana, and P. Sunshine, *Gastroenterology* **59**: 240 (1970).

129. J. J. Herbst and P. Sunshine, *Pediat. Res.* **3**: 27 (1969).

130. J. J. Herbst, and O. Koldovský, *Biochem. J.* **126**: 471 (1972).

131. J. J. Herbst, P. Sunshine, and N. Kretchmer, Intestinal Malabsorption in Infancy and Childhood, *Adv. Pediatr.* **16**: 11 (1969).

132. A. Heringová, V. Jirsová, and O. Koldovský, *Canad. J. Biochem.* **43**: 173 (1965).

133. A. Heringová, O. Koldovský, V. Jirsová, J. Uher, R. Noack, H. Friedrich, and G. Schenk, *Gastroenterology* **51**: 1023 (1966).

134. A. Heringová, C. S. Catz, J. Krasner, M. R. Juchau, and S. J. Yaffe, *Proc. Soc. Exptl. Biol. Med.* **127**: 875 (1968a).

135. A. Heringová, O. Koldovský, S. J. Yaffe, and V. Jirsová, *Biol. Neonat.* **13**: 1 (1968).

136. A. Heringová, O. Koldovský, S. J. Yaffe, V. Jirsová, and J. Uher, *Biol. Neonat.* **14**, 265 (1969).

137. H. J. Herschel, W. B. Hill, and J. W. B. Porter, *Proc. Nutr. Soc.* **201**: (1961).

138. L. A. Herzenberg and L. A. Herzenberg, *Nutr. Rev.* **17**: 65 (1959).

139. A. F. Hess, *Amer. J. Dis. Child.* **6**: 264 (1913).

140. K. J. Hill, *Quart. J. Exptl. Med.* **41**: 421 (1956).

141. K. J. Hill and W. S. Hardy, *Nature* **178**: 1353 (1956).

142. W. A. Hilton, *Amer. J. Physiol.* **1**: 459 (1902).

143. A. F. Hofmann, and B. Borgström, *Fed. Proc.* **21**: 44 (1962).

144. A. F. Hofmann and B. Borgström, *J. Clin. Invest.* **43**: 247 (1964).

145. D. E. Hogue, R. G. Warner, C. H. Griffin, and J. K. Loosli, *J. Anim. Sci.* **15**: 788 (1956).

146. F. Howard, and J. Yudkin, *Brit. J. Nutr.* **17**: 182 (1963).

147. D. Y. Y. Hsia, *Biochim. Biophys. Acta* **122**: 550 (1966).

148. J. T. Huber, N. L. Jacobson, R. S. Allen, and P. A. Hartman, *J. Dairy Sci.* **44**: 1494 (1961).

149. H. J. Huhtikangas, *Acta Soc. Med. Tenn* **24**: 1 (1936).

150. J. Husband, and P. Husband, *Lancet* ii: 409 (1969).

151. J. Husband, P. Husband, C. N. Mallinson *Lancet* i: 290 (1970).

152. J. Ibrahim, *Vers Ges. Dtsch. Naturforsch. Aerzte* **80**: 316 (1908).

153. J. Ibrahim, *Biochem. Z* **22**: 24 (1909).

154. E. C. Jarrett, and O. H. Hollman, *Arch. Dis. Child.* **41**: 525 (1966).

155. V. Jirsová, O. Koldovský, A. Heringová, and J. Hošková, *Biol. Neonat.* **8**: 30 (1965).

156. V. Jirsová, O. Koldovský, A. Heringová, J. Hošková, J. Jirásek, and J. Uher, *Biol. Neonat.* **9**: 44 (1966).

157. V. Jirsová, O. Koldovský, A. Heringová, J. Uher, and J. Jodl, *Biol. Neonat.* **13**: 143 (1968).

158. F. P. Johnson, *Amer. J. Anat.* **14**: 187 (1913).

159. S. M. Jordan, and E. H. Morgan, *Austr. J. Exptl. Biol. Med. Sci.* **46**: 465 (1968).

160. L. Josefsson, T. Lindberg, *Acta Physiol. Scand.* **66**: 410 (1966).

161. A. Kaeckenbeeck, M. El-Nageh, and F. Schoenae, *Amer. Med. Vet.* **61**: 391 (1967).

162. W. Kahn, *Kinderheilkinde* **33**: 48 (1922).

163. L. T. Kapralova, *Dokl. Akad Nauk USSR* **148**: 985 (1963).

164. M. F. L. Keene and E. F. Hewer, *Lancet* **1**: 767 (1929).

165. W. A. Kelly, *Nature* **186**: 97 (1960).

166. D. F. Kidder, M. J. Manners, and M. R. McCrea, *Res. Vet. Sci.* **21**: 227 (1961).

167. D. F. Kidder, M. J. Manners, M. R. McCrea, and A. D. Osborne, *Br. J. Nutr.* **22**: 501 (1968).

168. W. D. Kitts, C. B. Bailey, and A. J. Wood, *Canad. J. Agric. Sci.* **36**: 45 (1954).

169. T. G. Klumpp, and V. Neale, *Amer. J. Dis. Child.* **40**: 1215 (1930).

170. O. Koldovský, *Development of the Functions of the Small Intestine in Mammals and Man.* Basel: Karger, 1969.

171. O. Koldovský, *Digestion and Absorption During Development in* U. Stave (Ed.) *Physiology of the Perinatal Period.* New York: (Appleton-Century-Crofts, 1970.

172. O. Koldovský and P. Sunshine, unpublished.

173. O. Koldovský, P. Hahn, and J. Jiránek, *Čs. Fysiol.* **7**: 491 (1958).

174. O. Koldovský, P. Hahn, J. K. Tintěra, and J. Jiránek, *Čs. Fysiol* **8**: 211 (1959).

175. O. Koldovský, P. Hahn, V. Melichar, and M. Novák, *Čs Fysiol.* **11**: 450 (1962).

176. O. Koldovský, J. Danysz, E. Faltová, and P. Hahn, *Physiol. Bohemoslov.* **12**: 208 (1963).

177. O. Koldovský, P. Hahn, V. Melichar, M. Novák, P. Procházka, J. Rokos, and Z. Vacek, *Biochim. Biophys. Acta Library* **1**: 161 (1963).

178. O. Koldovský, H. Dominas, M. Muzyčenková, *Physiol. Bohemoslov.* **13**: 435 (1969).

179. O. Koldovský and F. Chytil, *Biochem. J.* **94**: 266 (1965).

180. O. Koldovský, V. Heringová, and V. Jirsová, *Physiol. Bohemoslov.* **14**: 228 (1965).

181. O. Koldovský, A. Heringová, V. Jirsová, J. E. Jirásek, and J. Uher, *Gastroenterology* **48**: 185 (1965b).

182. O. Koldovský, R. Noack, G. Schenk, V. Jirsová, A. Heringová, H. Braná, F. Chytil, and M. Friedrich, *Biochem. J.* **99**: 492 (1965).

183. O. Koldovský, A. Heringová, V. Jirsová, *Nature* **206**: 300 (1965).

184. O. Koldovský, A. Heringová, V. Jirsová, J. F. Jirásek, and J. Uher, *Canad. J. Biochem.* **44**: 523 (1966).

185. O. Koldovský, P. Sunshine, and N. Kretchmer, *Nature* **212**: 1389 (1966).

186. O. Koldovský, N-G, Asp, and A. Dahlqvist, *Analyt. Bioch.* **27**: 409 (1969).

187. O. Koldovský and J. Herbst, *Biology of Neonate.* **17**: 1 (1970).

188. O. Koldovský, J. Herbst, D. Burke, and P. Sunshine, *Growth* **34**: 359 (1970).

189. O. Koldovský and P. Sunshine, *Biochem. J.* **117:** 467 (1970).

190. B. Konopacka, *Folia morph.* **11:** 247 (1960).

191. C. S. Koshtoyants, Discussion in: *Development of Homeostasis*, London: Academic Press 1963, p. 213.

192. H. C. Koshtoyants, and R. D. Mitropolitanskaya, *Fiziol. Zhur. SSSR* **17:** 309 (1934).

193. H. C. Koshtoyants and R. D. Mitropolitanskaya, *Fiziol. Zhur. SSSR* **19:** 687 (1935).

194. K. Koštial, I. Šimonovič, M. Pišonič, *Nature* **215:** 1181 (1967).

195. J. P. Kraehenbuhl, E. Gloor, B. Blanc, Z. *Zellforschung* **76:** 170 (1967).

196. J. P. Kraehenbuhl and M. A. Campiche, *J. Cell. Biol.* **42:** 345 (1969).

197. A. P. Kryutschkova, *Fiziol. Zhur. USSR* **27:** 437 (1939).

198. K. Kubát and O. Koldovský, *Acta Histochem.* **33:** 75 (1969).

199. N. M. F. Leat and F. A. Harrison, *Biochem. J.* **105:** 13P (1967).

200. J. G. Lecce, *Biol. Neonat.* **9:** 50 (1966).

201. J. G. Lecce and E. Matrone, *J. Nutr.* **73:** 167 (1961).

202. J. G. Lecce, G. Matrone, and D. O. Morgan, *J. Nutr.* **73:** 158 (1961).

203. J. G. Lecce and D. O. Morgan, *J. Nutr.* **78:** 263 (1962).

204. J. G. Lecce, D. O. Morgan, and G. Matrone, *J. Nutr.* **84:** 43 (1964).

205. J. C. Leissring, and J. W. Anderson, *Amer. J. Anat.* **109:** 175 (1961).

206. J. C. Leissring, J. W. Anderson, and D. W. Smith, *Amer. J. Dis. Child.* **103:** 160 (1962).

207. F. W. Lengemann, *J. Nutr.* **99:** 419 (1969).

208. R. J. Levin, O. Koldovský, J. Hošková, V. Jirsová, and J. Uher, *Gut* **9:** 206 (1968).

209. J. Lieberman, *Gastroenterology* **50:** 183 (1966).

210. T. Lindberg, *Clin. Sci.* **30:** 505 (1966).

211. T. Lindberg and B. S. Karlsson, *Gastroenterology* **59:** 247 (1970).

212. T. Lindberg and Ch. Owman, *Acta Physiol. Scand.* **68:** 141 (1966).

213. L. E. Lloyd, E. W. Crampton, and V. G. McKay, *J. Anim. Sci.* **16:** 383 (1957).

214. L. F. Lloyd and C M. McCay, *J. Geront.* **10:** 182 (1955).

215. C. H. Long, D. E. Ullrey, E. R. Miller, *J. Anim. Sci.* **23:** 882 (1969).

216. G. Luther and K. Schreier, *Klin. Wschr.* **41:** 187 (1963).

217. S. Madey, and J. Dawis, *Pediat.* **4:** 177 (1949).

218. I. A. Manville, and R. W. Lloyd, *Amer. J. Physiol.* **100:** 394 (1932).

219. M. Masnerová, O. Koldovský, and K. Kubát, Experientia **25:** 518 (1966).

220. S. Mason, *Arch. Dis. Child.* **37:** 387 (1962).

221. J. H. Mason, T. Dalling, and W. S. Cordon, *J. Path. Bact.* **33:** 783 (1930).

222. N. Matsusaka and J. Inaba, *Nature* **214:** 303 (1967).

223. C. R. McLain, *Amer. J. Obstet. Gynecol.* **86:** 1079 (1963).

224. D. M. McMurphy, and L. O. Boréus, *Biol. Neonat.* **13:** 325 (1968).

225. N. Mechel, *Dtsch. Arch. Physiol.* **3:** 57 (1917).

226. V. Melichar, M. Novák, P. Hahn, O. Koldovský, and L. Zeman, *Acta Paediat.* **51**: 481 (1962).

227. V. Melichar, and M. Novák, in P. Hahn and O. Koldovský, (108).

228. W. F. Mengert, and J. W. Bourland, *Amer. J. Obstet. Gynecol.* **50**: 79 (1945).

229. T. G. Merrill, H. Sprinz, and A. J. Tousim, J. *Ultrastructure* **19**: 304 (1967).

230. F. Mignone and D. Castello, *Minerva Pediat.* **13**: 1098 (1961).

231. A. Miller, *Arch. Dis. Child.* **16**: 22 (1941).

232. P. F. Millington and P. W. A. Tovell, *Histochemical J.* **1**: 311 (1969).

233. S. D. Mistilis and P. Mearrick, *Gastroenterology* **58**: 286 (1970).

234. W. von Mollendorff, *Munch. Med. Woch.* **71**: 569 (1924).

235. F. Moog, *J. Exptl. Zool.* **118**: 187 (1951).

236. F. Moog, *J. Exptl. Zool.* **124**: 329 (1953).

237. F. Moog, *Developmental Biol.* **3**: 153 (1961).

238. F. Moog, *Fed. Proc.* **21**: 51 (1962).

239. F. Moog and V. Nehari, *Science* **119**: 809 (1954).

240. F. Moog and E. T. Thomas, *Endocrinology* **56**: 187 (1955).

241. B. Morris, *Proc. Roy. Soc.* (*London*), **B148**: 84 (1957).

242. B. Morris, *Proc. Roy. Soc.* (*London*), **B158**: 253 (1963).

243. B. Morris and E. D. Steel, *J. Endocrin.* **30**: 195 (1969).

244. I. G. Morris, Gamma Globulin Absorption in the Newborn, in *Handb. Physiol.*, Amer. Physiol. Soc. Section VI, **III**: 1491, (1968).

245. B. Mosinger, Z. Placer, and O. Koldovský, *Nature* **184**: 1245 (1959).

246. P. Nathan, *Fed. Proc.* **24**: 526 (1965).

247. H. Newey, *Brit. Med. Bull.* **23**: 236 (1967).

248. M. Ning, S. Reiser, and P. A. Christiansen, *Proc. Soc. Exptl. Biol. Med.* **129**: 799 (1968).

249. D. A. Nixon, and D. A. Wright, *Biol. Neonat.* **7**: 167 (1964).

250. R. Noack, O. Koldovský, M. Friedrich, A. Heringová, V. Jirsová, and G. Schenk, *Biochem. J.* **100**: 775 (1966).

251. R. Noack, G. Schenk, J. Proll, P. Hahn, O. Koldovský, *Biochem. Z.* **343**: 146 (1965).

252. C. Nordström, A. Dahlqvist, and L. Joseffson, *J. Histochem. Cytochem.* **15**: 713 (1967).

253. C. Nordström, O. Koldovský, and A. Dahlqvist, *J. Histochem. Cytochem.* **17**: 341 (1969).

254. C. Nordström, and A. Dahlqvist, *Biochim. Biophys. Acta* **198**: 621 (1970).

255. H. W. Oecklitz and B. Reinmuth, *Z. Kinderheilk* **82**: 321 (1959).

256. J. Overton, *J. Exptl. Zool.* **159**: 195 (1965).

257. C. H. Owman, *Quart. J. Exptl. Physiol.* **48**: 408 (1963).

258. D. Padaliková, *Zbl. Veterinaermed.* **13A**: 709 (1966).

259. D. B. Parrish and F. C. Fountain, *J. Dairy Sci.* **35**: 839 (1952).

260. V. Patzelt, Sitzungsber. der Wiener Akademie, *Math. Anat. Kl.* **86**: 145 (1882).

261. B. M. Patzelt, *Z. Mikr.-Anat. Forsch.* **27**: 269 (1931).

262. L. C. Payne and C. L. Marsh, *Fed. Proc.* **21**: 909 (1962).

263. L. C. Payne and C. L. Marsh, *J. Nutr.* **76**: 151 (1962).

264. H. Pelichová, O. Koldovský, J. Uher, J. Kraml, A. Heringová, and V. Jirsová, *Biol. Neonat.* **10**: 281 (1966).

265. A. Pelichová, O. Koldovský, A. Heringová, V. Jirsová, and J. Kraml, *Canad. J. Biochem.* **45**: 1375 (1967).

266. L. Perič-Golia and H. Sočič, *Amer. J. Physiol.* **215**: 1284 (1968).

267. R. A. Phillips and H. Gilder, *Endocrinology* **27**: 601 (1940).

268. A. E. Pierce and P. Johnson, *J. Hyg.* **58**: 247 (1960).

269. A. E. Pierce, P. C. Risdall, and B. Shaw, *J. Physiol.* **171**: 203 (1964).

270. A. E. Pierce and M. V. Smith, *J. Physiol.* **190**: 1 (1967).

271. A. E. Pierce and M. W. Smith, *J. Physiol.* **190**: 19 (1967).

272. N. Plimmer, *J. Physiol.* **35**: 20 (1906–7).

273. J. R. Poley, J. C. Dower, C. A. Owen, and G. B. Stickler, *J. Lab. Clin. Med.* **63**: 838 (1969); 43 (1964).

274. P. Procházka, P. Hahn, O. Koldovský, M. Nohýnek, and J. Rokos, *Physiol. Bohemoslov.* **13**: 208 (1964).

275. W. Reeve-Ramsey, *Jb. Kinkerheilk* **68**: 191 (1908).

276. S. Reiser, J. F. Fitzgerald, and P. A. Christiansen, *Biochim. Biophys. Acta* **203**: 351 (1970).

277. R. Rodewald, *J. Cell. Biol.* **45**: 635 (1970).

278. J. Rokos, P. Hahn, O. Koldovský, and P. Procházka, *Physiol. Bohemoslov.* **12**: 213 (1963).

279. P. Rosa, *Gynecol. Obstet.* **50**: 463 (1951).

280. L. Ross and E. B. Goldsmith, *Proc. Exptl. Biol. Med.* **90**: 56 (1955).

281. R. M. Rothberg, *J. Pediat.* **75**: 391 (1969).

282. A. Rubino, F. Zimbalatti, and S. Auriccho, *Biochim. Biophys. Acta* **92**: 305 (1964).

283. A. Rubino, M. Pierro, G. La Torreta, M. Vetrel, D. Di Martino, and S. Auricchio, *Pediat. Res.* **3**: 313 (1969).

284. P. Salenius, *Acta Anat.* **50**: Supplement 46 (1962).

285. M. Sámel and A. Čaputa, *Canad. J. Physiol. Pharmacol.* **43**: 431 (1965).

286. J. J. Sampson, *J. Biol. Chem.* **38**: 345 (1919).

287. W. Schmidt. *Z. Anat. Entwicklungsgeschicht* **126**: 276 (1967).

288. L. Schneider and J. Szathmary, *J. Immunforsch* **95**: 177 (1939).

289. R. D. Scow, and V. G. Foglia, *Amer. J. Physiol.* **166**: 541 (1951).

290. H. L. Segal and Y. S. Kim, *Proc. Natl. Acad. Sci.* (USA), **50**: 912 (1963).

291. A. Sesso, *Compt. Rend. Acad. Sci.* (*Paris*) **254**: 569, 1962.

292. A. D. Shannon and A. K. Lascelles, *Aust. J. Biol. Sci.* **19**: 831 (1966).

293. A. D. Shannon and A. K. Lascelles, *Aust. J. Biol. Sci.* **20**: 669 (1967).

294. A. D. Shannon and A. K. Lascelles, *J. Exp. Physiol.* **53**: 415 (1968).

295. A. D. Shannon and A. K. Lascelles, *Aust. J. Biol. Sci.* **22**: 189 (1969).

296. M. R. Sikov, J. M. Thomas, and D. D. Mahl, *Growth* **33**: 57 (1969).

297. R. Smallwood, R. Lester, A. S. Brown, G. J. Piasecki, and B. T. Jackson, Abstracts, 62nd Meeting of American Society for Clin. Invest., 1970, p. 900.

298. C. A. Smith, *The Physiology of the Newborn Infant*, 2nd ed. Springfield, Ill.: Thomas, 1953.

299. M. W. Smith and A. F. Pierce, *Nature* 213: 1150 (1967).

300. M. W. Smith, R. Witty, and P. Brown, *Nature* 220: 387 (1968).

301. R. H. Smith, *Nature* 198: 161 (1963).

302. T. Smith, *J. Exp. Med.* 41: 81 (1925).

303. K. Snoo, M Schr. Geburtsh. Gynak. 105: 88 (1937).

304. D. A. T. Southgate, E. M. Widdowson, B. J. Smits, W. T. Cooke, G. H. M. Walker, N. P. Walker, N. P. Mathers, *Lancet* i: 487 (1969).

305. H. Speert, *Amer. J. Obstet. Gynecol.* 45: 69 (1943).

306. L. M. Srivastava and G. Hübscher, *Biochem. J.* 110: 607 (1968).

307. B. States and S. Segal, *Biochim. Biophys. Acta* 163: 154 (1968).

308. F. Sterk, *Path. Microbiol.* 24: 963 (1961).

309. V. V. Steck and N. Kretchmer, *Pediat.* 34: 609 (1964).

310. P. Sunshine, and N. Kretchmer, *Science* 144: 850 (1969).

311. G. F. Sutherland, *Amer. J. Physiol.* 55: 398 (1921).

312. T. Tachibana, *Jap. J. Obstet.* 10: 40 (1927).

313. T. Tachibana, *Jap. J. Obstet.* 11: 92 (1928).

314. T. Tachibana, *Jap. J. Obstet.* 11: 227 (1928).

315. T. Tachibana, *Jap. J. Obstet.* 12: 21 (1929).

316. T. Tachibana, *Jap. J. Obstet.* 12: 39 (1929).

317. T. Tachibana, *Jap. J. Obstet.* 12: 100 (1929).

318. T. Tachibana, *Jap. J. Obstet.* 15: 27 (1932).

319. D. T. Taylor, P. H. Bligh, and M. H. Duggan, *Biochem. J.* 83: 25 (1962).

320. J. Thomson, *Arch. Dis. Child.* 26: 558 (1951).

321. J. D. Trasher, *Experientia* 23: 1050 (1967).

322. Ch. Tso-Kan, M. A. Hwei-Yun, *Acta Anat. Sinica* 8: 307 (1965).

323. J. P. Turchini, R. Pourmadi, and P. Malet, *C. R. Soc. Biol.* 159: 663 (1965).

324. Z. Vacek, *Čs. Morpol.* 12: 292 (1964).

325. Z. Vacek, P. Hahn, and O. Koldovský, *Čs. Morfol.* 12: 292 (1962).

326. J. H. Van DeKamer and H. A. Weijer, *5th Internat. Congr. Nutrition*, Panel paper 7, 19 (1960).

327. J. Verne, *Ann. Endocrinol. (Paris)* 12: 810 (1951).

328. J. Verne and S. Hebert, *Ann. Endocrinol. (Paris)* 10: 456 (1949).

329. J. Verne, S. Hebert, and O. Charpal, *C. R. Soc. Biol.* 146: 176 (1952).

330. J. Verne and S. Hebert, *Ann. Endocrinol. (Paris)* 17: 413 (1956).

331. R. G. Vernon and D. G. Walker, *Biochem. J.* 118: 531 (1970).

332. R. Verzár and E. J. McDougall, *Absorption from the Intestine*. London: Longmans, Green, 1936.

333. L. Vollrath, *Z. Zellforschung* 50: 36 (1959).

334. L. Vollrath, *Adv. Anat. Embryol. Cell. Biol.* 41: 2 (1969).

335. H. Wagner, *Biol. Neonat.* **3:** 257 (1961).

336. D. M. Walker, *J. Agr. Sci.* **52:** 357, 374 (1959).

337. N. Weinland, *Z. Biol.* **38:** 16 (1899).

338. H. Welsh, F. Heinz, G. Lagally, and K. Stuhlfauth, *Klin. Wchschr.* **43:** 902 (1965).

339. J. D. Welsh and A. Walker, *Proc. Soc. Exptl. Biol. Med.* **120:** 525 (1965).

340. N. Werner, *Acta Pediat.* **35:** suppl. 6 (1948).

341. H. G. K. Westenbrink, *Arch. Né~erl* **21:** 18 (1936).

342. E. M. Widdowson, *Lancet* **27:** 1099 (1965).

343. D. L. Williams G. H. Spray, *J. Nutr.* **22:** 297 (1968).

344. R. M. Williams and F. Beck, *Histochem. J.* **1:** 531 (1969).

345. R. M. Williams and F. Beck, *J. Anat.* **105:** 487 (1969).

346. D. H. Wilson and E. C. C. Lin, *Amer. J. Physiol.* **199:** 1030 (1960).

347. W. F. Windle and C. L. Bishop, *Proc. Soc. Exptl. Biol.* **40:** 2 (1939).

348. S. F. Wissig and D. O. Graney, *J. Cell. Biol.* **39:** 564 (1968).

349. G. H. Wright and D. A. Nixon, *Nature* **190:** 816 (1961).

350. N. Yanose, *Pflügers Arch. Gen. Physiol.* **1171:** 345 (1907).

351. K. Znamenáček, and H. Přibylová, *Čs. pediat.* **18:** 104 (1963).

352. J. Zoula, V. Melichar, M. Novák, P. Hahn, and O. Koldovský, *Acta Pediat.* **55:** 26 (1966).

# 6

## Metabolic Changes in Children with Protein-Calorie Malnutrition

G. A. O. ALLEYNE, H. FLORES, D. I. M. PICOU,
and J. C. WATERLOW

Medical Research Council, Tropical Metabolism Research Unit, University of the
West Indies, Kingston 7, Jamaica

As we write in 1970 it is probably still true to say that protein-calorie malnutrition (PCM) in infants and young children is the most serious health problem with which the world is faced (Bengoa, 11). Malnutrition, in principle, is preventable, but efficient prevention and effective cure require a better understanding of the underlying processes.

In the last decade a great deal of work has been devoted in many centers throughout the world to studying the biochemical and metabolic changes that occur in PCM. It is impossible in one chapter to do justice to all the valuable contributions that have been made. The subject was reviewed in detail by Viteri et al. (133) in 1964, and therefore we have concentrated on work done since that date. We have also confined ourselves almost entirely to studies on human subjects, since it is impossible over such a wide field to touch even briefly on all the relevant animal experiments. Finally, we recognize that it is artificial to treat changes in metabolism in isolation from other types of change, e.g., in endocrine activity or in body and cell composition, but this is a practical limitation that has to be accepted.

Since *kwashiorkor* and *marasmus* are mentioned frequently in the sections that follow, a word must be said about the meaning of these names. They are conventional terms, based on clinical characteristics, which unfortunately are used by different people in different ways.

Throughout the world it is accepted that the distinguishing feature of kwashiorkor is oedema. Some authors require one or more specific changes to be present before they make the diagnosis (e.g., changes in skin, mucosae or hair, and hepatomegaly). For others oedema alone is sufficient. The characteristic of the marasmic child is severe wasting of muscle and subcutaneous tissue without oedema or other specific signs.

These are the two typical forms, often described as the two ends of the spectrum, but they are not necessarily the commonest. The prevailing type varies from one region of the world to another. In some places mixed pictures are most frequent; for example, severe wasting with slight oedema or hepatomegaly. There are, of course, differences in severity as well as in clinical picture. Many authors by convention have restricted the term *marasmus* to children who are less than 60% of the expected weight for age according to the Boston standards (Nelson, 82). This corresponds to "third degree malnutrition" in the classification of Gomez et al. (41).

In this chapter, when different authors are quoted, we have preserved unchanged the names they have used. Some of the discrepancies that exist between observations from different parts of the world may arise from imperfections of nomenclature that disguise real and important differences. The 3-year old child with kwashiorkor in Guatemala is not necessarily the same as the 1-year old in Jamaica. Similarly, the term *marasmic* has been applied equally to the *nutritional dwarfs* in Chile who are not clinically ill and to patients with gastroenteritis and malnutrition in Jamaica who are very severely ill.

In Jamaica we have found rather few clear-cut biochemical or metabolic differences between patients with kwashiorkor and marasmus, and in any case in this region mixed or intermediate forms are commonest. Frequently, therefore, all malnourished children have been treated as a single group.

## CARBOHYDRATE METABOLISM

An increasing interest has been shown in carbohydrate metabolism in infantile malnutrition. Studies have ranged from investigations into the absorption of sugars and their effect on intestinal function to attempts at dissecting the pathways of carbohydrate metabolism in tissues such as liver and muscle. Efforts are also being made to define in biochemical terms the defects in energy production which must underlie the apathy and weakness characteristic of the malnourished child.

## Absorption of Sugars

Dean in Uganda (30) noted that in some children with kwashiorkor diarrhoea worsened when they were fed milk and attributed this condition to some abnormality of carbohydrate absorption. Trowell, Davies, and Dean (126) also showed that there was a specific intolerance of lactose. Subsequent studies have focused on the enzyme defects in the intestine and the osmotic effects of the failure to absorb sugars. It is now clear that many children with kwashiorkor have low levels of the enzymes lactase, sucrase, and maltase in their intestinal mucosa (Bowie et al. 17; James, 58). Bowie et al. showed that a lactose-containing diet led to an increase in stool weight with large amounts of lactic acid in the stool. This lactose intolerance could persist even after one year on an adequate diet.

James (58A) has used the intestinal perfusion technique to show that there may be impaired absorption not only of lactose and sucrose but also of monosaccharides. Some typical data are given in Table 1,

**Table 1    The Rate of Absorption of Sugar from a 40-Cm Length of Jejunum in 10 Children before and after Recovery from Malnutrition**

| Sugar infused | Glucose | Glucose | Glucose | Lactose | Sucrose |
|---|---|---|---|---|---|
| Rate of infusion (mmole/hr) | 12.5 | 25 | 50 | 25 | 26.3 |
| Mean rate of absorption, (mmole/hr) | | | | | |
| Malnourished | 7.4 | 11.0 | 16.0 | 7.3 | 11.6 |
| Treated | 9.6 | 19.4 | 33.7 | 15.4 | 18.2 |
| $P$ | $>0.05$ | $<0.005$ | $<0.005$ | $<0.0025$ | $>0.05$ |

which shows clearly the poor absorption with lactose infusions (James 58A). In parallel biopsy studies it was found that the rate of absorption correlated well with the level of intestinal disaccharidase activity.

## Blood Glucose Levels and Glucose Tolerance

There are widely different reports on the effect of malnutrition on blood glucose levels. Workers in South Africa (Sloane et al., 115), Nigeria (Baig and Edozien, 9), Chile (Oxman et al., 86), Jordan (Hopkins et al., 57), Uganda (Whitehead and Harland, 150), Jamaica (Alleyne and Scullard, 4, and James and Coore, 60) have all found that malnourished children have low levels of blood glucose. As Table 2 shows,

**Table 2  Fasting Levels of Blood Glucose in Malnourished Children from Different Countries**

| Authors | Country | Clinical type | Blood glucose (mg%; mean or range) |
|---|---|---|---|
| Sloane et al. | South Africa | Kwashiorkor | 51 |
| Aballi | Cuba | Marasmus | 71 |
| Baig and Edozien | Nigeria | Kwashiorkor | 65 |
| Oxman et al. | Chile | Marasmus | 55 |
| Whitehead and Harland | Uganda | Kwashiorkor | 31–69 |
| Kerpel-Fronius | Hungary | Marasmus | 0–102 |
|  |  | Kwashiorkor | 45–100 |
| James and Coore | Jamaica | Marasmic/kwashiorkor | 52 |
| Flores et al. | Jamaica | Marasmic/kwashiorkor | 53 |

however, there is much variation in the degree of hypoglycaemia; Whitehead and Harland (150) record several patients with blood glucose level below 40 mg%. A serious consequence is that dangerously low levels of blood sugar may be present without any of the usual symptoms. On the other side, there are reports from South Africa (Bowie, 16) and Peru (Graham et al., 42) which show that malnourished children may have normal or slightly elevated blood sugar concentrations.

There is also variation in the results of glucose tolerance tests. Sloane et al. (115), Baig and Edozien (9), Hadden (43), and Bowie (16), all working in Africa, showed that there is impairment of glucose tolerance in patients with kwashiorkor, but the last two workers claim that in marasmic infants tolerance is normal. This is in direct contrast to studies in Chile, where Oxman et al. (86) reported marked glucose intolerance in marasmic infants. If there is a difference in calorie intake between the two clinical groups, it is not unlikely that there will be differences in glucose tolerance. Perhaps even the nature of the preceding calorie intake is of importance.

Impaired glucose utilization may be related directly to cell damage in the pancreatic islets, thus causing reduced release of insulin in response to a glucose load, or there may be peripheral insensitivity to insulin. Plasma insulin levels are generally low in malnutrition (Baig and Edozien, 9; James and Coore, 60; Hadden, 43; Milner, 77) and there is little or no rise after intravenous glucose. This would suggest that the cause of the carbohydrate intolerance is the poor response of the cells of the pancreas. Bowie (16) has reported, however, that intravenous injection of insulin (0.25 units/kg) did not improve the glucose tolerance of patients with kwashiorkor. Pimstone and coworkers (Pimstone et al., 90–92) found increased levels of growth hormone in the serum in malnutrition; cortisol levels are also raised (Alleyne and Young, 2; Rao et al., 98). Both effects would tend to decrease the sensitivity to insulin. By analogy with other clinical situations, such as acromegaly or Cushing's syndrome, it is highly likely that these hormones do play a part in producing glucose intolerance.

Hopkins et al. (57) have attributed glucose intolerance in malnutrition to chromium deficiency. In a study in Jordan and Nigeria they showed that in areas in which there is a low concentration of chromium in the drinking water glucose intolerance was more pronounced. They claimed that oral administration of chromium led to marked improvement after only one day of treatment. The biochemical basis of this hypothesis is not clear, and Carter et al. (21) failed to confirm the effect of chromium in Egyptian patients with kwashiorkor.

It is doubtful if there are any severe immediate effects of glucose intolerance in malnourished children, but it is obviously important to know whether it improves or whether it persists into later life and predisposes to frank diabetes mellitus. Baig and Edozien (9) were able to follow their patients after treatment and found a progressive improvement. Hadden (43) showed that there was a return to normal by the fourteenth day of treatment. On the other hand, James and Coore (60) in Jamaica found that glucose tolerance was still impaired even when the children had apparently recovered completely and had approached their ideal weight for their height (Table 3). In the initial stages no differences were observed between patients with the clinical features of kwashiorkor or marasmus, and therefore they have been treated as a single group.

In the longest follow up yet reported Cook (27) examined children who had been treated for kwashiorkor 6 to 12 years before; he found that there was still a significant impairment of glucose tolerance. Cook's findings are all the more important when it is appreciated that his controls were children from the same environment who presumably were having the same diet as the test subjects.

Table 3   Blood Glucose Levels and the Rate of
Glucose Disappearance after Intravenous Injection
in Malnourished and Recovered Children

|  | Fasting Blood Glucose (mg/100 ml) | $K^a$ (%/min) |
|---|---|---|
| Malnourished | $45.0 \pm 2.7$ | $1.95 \pm 0.11$ |
| Recovered | $70.6 \pm 1.7$ | $2.53 \pm 0.16$ |
| Normal | $74.0 \pm 2.7$ | $3.45 \pm 0.36$ |

[a] $K$ is the slope of the disappearance curve plotted semi-logarithmically against time.


### Glycolysis and Gluconeogenesis

Attention is beginning to be directed toward the functioning of some of the known pathways of carbohydrate metabolism in malnutrition. Whitehead and Harland (150) reported elevated levels of lactate and pyruvate in blood from patients with kwashiorkor and suggested the presence of a block in the entry of pyruvate into the Krebs cycle, such as occurs in deficiencies of vitamins $B_1$ or $B_{12}$ (Buckle, 19). Oxman et al. (86) also showed that blood pyruvate levels in marasmic infants were higher than normal and did not rise after intravenous injection of glucose. In Jamaica malnourished children were found to have normal fasting levels of pyruvate and lactate (Alleyne and Scullard, 3); in contrast to recovered children the levels did not rise after glucose was given intravenously, thus confirming the findings of Oxman. This result suggests that there may be an impairment of glycolysis.

Metcoff et al. (76) measured metabolic intermediates as well as the enzyme pyruvate kinase in muscle biopsy samples from malnourished children and found decreased levels of phosphoenol pyruvate and oxaloacetate but normal levels of pyruvate. The activity of pyruvate kinase was reduced and evidence was obtained of a change in the kinetic properties of the enzyme when it was assayed in vitro with substrates and cofactors at concentrations similar to those that exist in the muscle of malnourished children. It is difficult to explain why in malnutrition the level of phosphoenol pyruvate should be low and that of pyruvate unchanged if in vivo there was a block at the level of pyruvate kinase. On the contrary, if levels of metabolic intermediates reflect the in vivo situation, the opposite change might be expected. A decrease in activity of pyruvate kinase and a reduction in ATP, pyruvate, and oxaloacetate have also been described in leucocytes of severely malnourished children (Yoshida et al., 156, 157). These authors also suggested a block of glycolysis at the terminal step with consequent reduction in ATP formation and impaired energy production.

If a block in glycolysis were a general phenomenon in malnutrition, this would be a good explanation of the glucose intolerance observed. On this hypothesis samples of muscle obtained from malnourished children might show impaired glycolysis in vitro. To test this Trust et al. (127) made homogenates of muscle biopsy samples and measured anaerobic lactate production from various substrates in malnourished children before and after recovery and in normal children who had never been malnourished. Lactate production from all substrates was essentially the same in malnourished and recovered children, but the values for both groups were lower than in normal children with two substrates—glucose-6-phosphate and fructose-1,6-diphosphate (Table 4).

**Table 4  Lactate Production *in vitro* by Muscle Samples from Malnourished, Recovered, and Normal Children**[a]

|  | Micro moles of Lactate per Gram of Alkali Soluble Protein per 30 Minutes | | |
|---|---|---|---|
|  | Malnourished (8) | Recovered (8) | Normal (5) |
| No substrate | $88 \pm 11.2$ | $96 \pm 15.6$ | $82 \pm 17.8$ |
| Glucose | $91 \pm 9.9$ | $97 \pm 16.0$ | $78 \pm 11.8$ |
| Glucose-6-phosphate | $195 \pm 36.6$ | $179 \pm 28.2$ | $418 \pm 87.6$ |
| Fructose-1,6-diphosphate | $166 \pm 17.5$ | $188 \pm 22.2$ | $305 \pm 23.6$ |
| Phosphoenolpyruvate | $110 \pm 14.1$ | $121 \pm 13.9$ | $136 \pm 24.0$ |

[a] Mean $\pm$ S.E.M. Number of patients in parentheses.

These preliminary findings suggest that there may be a block in glycolysis distal to fructose-1,6-diphosphate, which persists even after clinical recovery.

### Gluconeogenesis

There is some evidence of enhanced hepatic gluconeogenesis in malnutrition (Alleyne and Scullard, 3). The increase in plasma cortisol and the decrease in plasma insulin would facilitate gluconeogenesis (Weber et al., 143). Our finding (see below) of increased levels of glucose-6-

phosphatase, a key enzyme of hepatic gluconeogenesis, would fit this picture. Additional evidence that there may be increased gluconeogenesis comes from studies in which labeled substrates have been infused, followed by measurement of incorporation of the label into other substrates. Gillman et al. (39) infused $^{14}C$ glucose, $^{14}C$ pyruvate and 1-$^{14}C$ acetate into children with kwashiorkor and showed that the complete oxidation of glucose was depressed. There was, however, a more ready synthesis of glucose from pyruvate in the malnourished infants. Synthesis of glucose from pyruvate involves first conversion of pyruvate to oxaloacetate by the enzyme pyruvate carboxylase (Shrago and Lardy, 114). If this step is indeed enhanced, it is unlikely that there could be an elevation of blood pyruvate caused by a block of entry of pyruvate into the Krebs cycle, as suggested by Whitehead and Harland (150).

Changes in plasma amino acids in relation to diet and gluconeogenesis have recently been extensively studied in adult man. Starvation causes a fall in plasma alanine, whereas a protein free diet produces a marked rise (Adibi, 1; Young and Scrimshaw, 158). It has been postulated that the level of plasma alanine may reflect the degree of hepatic gluconeogenesis (31).

In infantile malnutrition the changes in plasma alanine concentration are not particularly striking (e.g., Holt et al., 56; Saunders et al., 108). This may be because there is usually a combined deficiency of both protein and calories.

Whitehead and Dean (149) showed that in kwashiorkor the properties of nonessential amino acids in the plasma (N/E ratio) is increased; this change is not seen, or is much less marked, in marasmus (Saunders et al., 108). Swendseid et al. (123) pointed out that in severe obesity and in some cases of diabetes the plasma N/E ratio is reduced. These conditions are associated with a high rate of gluconeogenesis, and Swendseid suggested that a low N/E ratio might be indicative of increased gluconeogenesis. From this evidence it might be supposed that gluconeogenesis is increased in marasmus, presumably at the expense of protein, but not in kwashiorkor, in which the dietary supply of carbohydrate is more nearly adequate.

In general it is probable that changes in plasma amino acids, which have hitherto been viewed as a reflection of changes in protein metabolism, may throw further light on the state of carbohydrate metabolism.

### Metabolism of Glycogen in Liver

If fasting blood sugar levels are low in malnutrition yet gluconeogenesis is active, there remains the possibility of impaired glycogenolysis. Earlier

histological and chemical assessments of liver glycogen in biopsy specimens gave inconsistent results (Waterlow and Weisz, 139; Salazar de
Souza, 106; Stuart et al., 122). Liver glycogen has been restudied in
Jamaica under carefully controlled conditions (Alleyne and Scullard,
3) and was found to be significantly reduced in the malnourished children (Table 5).

**Table 5   Glycogen Concentration and Glucose-6-Phosphatase
Activity in the Liver in Malnutrition[a]**

|  | Glycogen (mg/100 mg wet wt) | Glucose-6-Phosphatase (units/100 mg protein) |
| --- | --- | --- |
| Malnourished | 2.02 ± 0.28 (18) | 4.85 ± 0.64 (14) |
| Recovering | 4.58 ± 0.88 (12) | 2.47 ± 0.23 (11) |
| Recovered | 5.85 ± 0.50 (13) | 2.98 ± 0.27 (14) |

[a] Mean ± S.E.M. Number of patients in parentheses. Glucose-6-phos-
phatase units = mg $P_i$ released per 15 minutes. Data of Alleyne and
Scullard (3), reproduced by courtesy of the Editor of *Clinical Science*.

Glucose-6-phosphatase is the final enzyme in the pathway of glucose
production, whether by gluconeogenesis or glycogenolysis. There is a
conflict of evidence about the effect of malnutrition on the activity of
this enzyme in the liver. Fletcher (32) found it to be reduced in malnourished infants and drew an analogy between malnutrition and Van
Gierke's disease (glycogenosis i) in which there is hypoglycaemia, increased liver glycogen, and low levels or absence of glucose-6-phospha-
tase. A reduction in glucose-6-phosphatase was also found in kwashiorkor
by Salazar de Souza (106) and Mukherjee and Noth (80). The latter
authors found normal levels of the enzyme in marasmic infants. Our
results showed that hepatic glucose-6-phosphatase activity was higher
in the malnourished child (Table 5); with recovery there was an increase
in liver glycogen and a decrease in glucose-6-phosphatase (Alleyne and
Scullard, 3). In a detailed study of the efficiency of hepatic glycogenolysis and the functional capacity of glucose-6-phosphatase we measured
blood glucose, lactate, and pyruvate after intravenous injection of glucagon. There was a prompt rise in blood glucose in all children, but in
those who had recovered the peak level was higher. Milner (77) obtained similar results. In addition, there was no significant rise in lactate
or pyruvate after glucagon in either group. After intravenous injection
of galactose blood glucose rose normally. The activity of liver phos-

phorylase was unaltered in the malnourished children. These findings, taken together, indicate that in our patients there was no significant impairment of glycogenolysis and glucose-6-phosphatase activity was adequate. Whitehead and Harland (150) also gave glucagon to patients with kwashiorkor and found that the increment in blood glucose was much lower than in children who had recovered. This could mean that there was a lower liver glycogen in their malnourished patients or that glycogenolysis was indeed impaired. These possibilities will have to be resolved by future work.

### Glycogen Metabolism in Muscle

The introduction of the muscle biopsy needle* described by Nichols et al. (83) and the development of microtechniques have opened up new possibilities for studies on muscle, which has a key role in the metabolism of carbohydrate and protein. Studies on muscle glycogen have been done in Jamaica and Guatemala (Alleyne and Scullard, 4; Alleyne et al., 5; Nichols et al., 84; Besterman and Alleyne, 14). The glycogen content of muscle is low in malnutrition and rises with recovery (Table 6). After the malnourished child has been on a good diet for

Table 6  Muscle Glycogen, Phosphorylase and Glycogen Synthetase at Varying Times During Recovery from Malnutrition[a]

| Days after admission | 1–3 | 7–9 | 21–27 | Recovered |
|---|---|---|---|---|
| Glycogen (g/100 g wet wt) | 0.14 (7) ± .056 | 1.21 (14) ± .223 | 1.88 (13) ± .166 | 0.98 (28) ± .075 |
| Total phosphorylase ($\mu$moles $P_i$/100 mg protein-min) | 9.7 (4) ±2.9 | 24.7 (5) ±9.4 | 63.3 (7) ±11.5 | 62.2 (19) ±6.9 |
| Total glycogen synthetase (counts incorporated /mg protein-min) | 233 (5) ±65 | 242 (7) ±44 | 478 (8) ±103 | 691 (9) ±108 |

[a] Mean ± S.E.M. Number of patients in parentheses.

approximately one week muscle glycogen rises to normal levels and after three weeks overshoots to values about twice the normal (Alleyne

* We are indebted to Dr. B. L. Nichols of the Children's Hospital, Houston, Texas for the gift of these needles.

and Scullard, 4; Besterman and Alleyne, 14). Muscle glycogen not only constitutes a carbohydrate reserve but perhaps by its osmotic effect serves to bind electrolytes, mainly potassium, intracellularly. There is a close correlation between the concentrations of potassium and glycogen in muscle (Alleyne et al., 5). There is no evidence, however, that when the overshoot of muscle glycogen occurs there is a similar increase in muscle potassium. It is possible that potassium deficiency may contribute to the initial low levels of glycogen in muscle.

In an attempt to detect changes in enzyme activity which might be related to these changes in muscle glycogen Besterman and Alleyne (14) measured phosphorylase and glycogen synthetase. There was no significant change in either enzyme after the child had been treated for one week, although during this time muscle glycogen concentration increased eightfold. Thereafter there were similar increases in both enzymes as the children recovered. Phosphorylase A was approximately 30% of the total phosphorylase at all stages. During the early phases of treatment the I form of glycogen synthetase (glucose-6-phosphate independent) bore a constant relationship to the D form of the enzyme (glucose-6-phosphate dependent), but when the children were fully recovered glycogen synthetase I was increased. This may be related to the increasing levels of insulin found during recovery. These changes have been interpreted as showing that the increase in glycogen is mediated mainly by increased availability of substrate without any detectable rise in enzyme activity. The only similar situation so far described in man was produced by depletion of muscle glycogen by exercise, followed by introduction of a high-carbohydrate diet. Muscle glycogen immediately rose to levels much higher than normal (Bergstrom and Hultman, 12). No enzymes were measured in that study.

Adrenaline can cause glycogenolysis in liver and muscle, although at the levels usually used in clinical studies it is mainly muscle glycogen that is broken down. Whitehead and Harland (150) found that after adrenaline was injected subcutaneously there was a poor hyperglycaemic response in patients with kwashiorkor. Rao (95) obtained similar data from his children with kwashiorkor, but it was remarkable that the rise in blood glucose was greater in those children who were marasmic than in those who had recovered from malnutrition.

### Animal Experiments

The most important work in this area has come from Heard and his colleagues (Stewart and Heard, 129; Heard et al., 50; Heard, 48; Heard and Turner, 49; Heard and Henry, 51, 52) who have investigated the effects of protein and calorie deficiency on glucose metabolism in pigs and dogs. Their results show the effect of species differences and also the importance of age in assessing the effects of malnutrition on glucose metabolism. Heard and coworkers claim that one effect of malnutrition is to cause delay in maturation of the processes that normally metabolize glucose. Young pigs have a relatively low glucose tolerance, and this effect is reproduced by protein deficiency. In protein-deficient pigs there was an increase in liver glycogen and decreased activity of glucose-6-phosphatase. An important point was that the levels of glucose-6-phosphatase were lower if the nutritional insult took place very early in life. Muscle glycogen was normal. These authors have also shown a close relationship between glucose tolerance and insulin sensitivity in pigs, but it tends to disappear with malnutrition when sensitivity to insulin progressively decreases. In dogs protein deficiency also caused impairment of glucose tolerance. In contrast with the pigs some relation between glucose tolerance and insulin sensitivity was still retained.

Rao (96) has reported on the effects of protein malnutrition on hepatic glycogen metabolism in rats. A low-protein, low-calorie diet led to an increase in liver glycogen. When only protein was restricted, glycogen levels increased in liver but decreased in muscle. The activity of hepatic glucose-6-phosphatase decreased in the livers of animals deprived of calories and protein.

## General Conclusion

The majority of studies show that malnutrition in children produces some reduction in blood glucose and an impairment of glucose tolerance. The cause of the hypoglycaemia is not obvious, but it may be related partly to impaired intestinal absorption. Glucose intolerance is reflected in poor lactate production following intravenous glucose. The results of the experiments in which muscle lactate production was measured in vitro, showing no difference between malnourished and recovered children, would indicate that the glucose intolerance is caused by poor transport of glucose into the cell rather than by any differences in enzyme activity along the glycolytic pathway. This may well be related to the poor insulin response to intravenous glucose. There is no evidence of impaired hepatic glycogenolysis, and muscle glycogen, although low initially, rises to normal and even supranormal levels with treatment. The animal experiments show that there is no single model that accurately reflects the human situation. There is, however, some indication that impaired glucose tolerance may resemble a state of delayed maturation of the normal processes of carbohydrate disposal.

The possibility that glucose intolerance may persist after apparent clinical recovery makes long-term studies necessary.


## LIPID METABOLISM

Up to 50% of the wet weight of the liver in kwashiorkor may be fat. Although chemical determinations in biopsy or autopsy specimens have been performed only occasionally, the high incidence of fatty infiltration of the liver is one of the best documented alterations of metabolism in kwashiorkor and is commonly used to differentiate it from the other type of infantile malnutrition, marasmus.

The attention of investigators in this field has been concentrated on two main questions: the origin of the excess liver fat and the mechanism of the fatty infiltration.


### The Origin of the Liver Fat

It is generally accepted that the aetiological difference between marasmus and kwashiorkor is the caloric intake, the protein intake being deficient in both cases. Thus it seems tempting to associate the relatively high caloric intake in kwashiorkor with the high incidence of fatty liver in this type of malnutrition, a relationship supported by animal experiments (Platt et al., 93).

The composition of the excess liver fat has been studied only exceptionally. Macdonald (70) found that up to 95% of the total liver lipids in children dying of malnutrition was in the fatty acid fraction. The lack of control values did not permit comparisons, but it has been accepted since then that triglycerides constitute the major lipid fraction in the liver in kwashiorkor; this has been confirmed by direct analysis of liver triglycerides in biopsy specimens: in Jamaican children levels up to 500 mg of triglycerides per gram of liver have been found (Seakins and Flores, 113, unpublished data).

The total phospholipid content of the liver falls within the range of values obtained from control children if expressed on the basis of fat-free weight (Chatterjee and Mukherjee, 24). These authors, however, found a reduction in the relative content of phosphatidylethanolamine, the significance of which is not yet understood. On the whole it appears that apart from the increased concentration of triglycerides the composition of the liver lipid is close to normal.

Despite the agreement that liver fat in kwashiokor must be derived from dietary calories, consisting mainly of carbohydrates, it is not certain whether the lipids are synthesized in the liver itself or reach it from the adipose tissue. One approach to this problem has been the study of the proportions of different fatty acids in liver and depot lipids. Baker and Macdonald (10) and Macdonald (71) found that the fatty acid patterns in both tissues were similar, the implication being that liver fat was derived from the adipose tissue. From essentially similar data, however, Macdonald et al. (72) later drew the opposite conclusion that liver fat was synthesized *in situ*. On the basis of the same experimental results Lewis et al. (68) again proposed fat depots as the source of liver lipids. They pointed out that both the release and uptake of fatty acids by the tissues are selective processes and that minor differences in the patterns of liver and adipose tissue need not invalidate their hypothesis. This experimental approach, which seems to be the only one employed so far, has led to divergent conclusions, and the results are difficult to interpret.

### The Mechanism of the Fatty Liver

Several hypotheses have been suggested to explain the pathogenesis of the fatty infiltration of the liver in kwashiorkor. Observations by different workers on lipid metabolism in this group of malnourished children have agreed remarkably well, with few exceptions, although the conclusions drawn from the data have been different.

A deficiency of essential fatty acids as contributory to the accumulation of fat in the liver has been suggested by Bronte-Stewart (18). Schendel and Hansen (109) observed a pattern of fatty acids in serum from patients recovering from kwashiorkor similar to that of a deficiency of essential fatty acids. They interpreted this to be the result of a great demand produced by increased mobilization of lipids rather than a real deficiency. This view is in agreement with a later study (Macdonald, 72) in which no significant changes were found in the pattern of essential fatty acids in liver during recovery from kwashiorkor.

The possibility of a specific deficiency of lipotropic factors was first considered by Waterlow (135). He administered choline, methionine, or inositol as dietary supplements to infants being treated for kwashiorkor, with no beneficial effects, as judged from serial histological analysis of liver biopsies or from the clinical estimation of liver size. These observations are in agreement with the finding of a normal concentration of liver phospholipids when allowance is made for the excess of liver triglycerides (Chatterjee and Mukherjee, 24). Moreover, total serum phospholipids are only slightly reduced in untreated patients and their rise during recovery is of little significance (Schwartz and Dean, 112;

Macdonald, 72; Lewis et al., 68; Flores et al., 33; Truswell and Hansen, 128; Truswell et al., 130).

Fletcher (32) reported a decrease in the activity of glucose-6-phosphatase in liver biopsies from children with kwashiorkor. This led to the suggestion that the inability to secrete glucose would enhance lipogenesis in the liver. This author also showed that liver biopsies could convert acetate into fatty acids in vitro; this synthetic activity, however, was the same in malnourished and recovered children, although the great scattering of the values makes the drawing of any conclusions impossible. Alleyne and Scullard (4), working with similar clinical material, have not been able to confirm the low glucose-6-phosphatase activity in the liver. Therefore the evidence for increased liver lipogenesis relies only on the observation of the fatty acid patterns of liver and fat depots, which, as shown, are difficult to interpret.

Lewis et al. (68) believed that the excess liver fat derives from an increased mobilization of free fatty acids from the depots. The evidence of increased levels of free fatty acids in serum in kwashiorkor is indeed quite consistent in several reports (Lewis et al., 68, 69; Fletcher, 32; Hadden, 43; Milner, 77). Fatty liver, however, can develop in children with normal levels of serum NEFA (Flores et al., 33), and high levels have also been reported in marasmus, in which fatty liver does not occur (Lewis et al., 68, 69; Milner, 77). Vomiting and diarrhoea are consistently reported as accompanying features of kwashiorkor. The stress and physiological starvation produced by both could explain the high levels of free fatty acids which may not necessarily need to be associated with fatty liver.

As mentioned above, the main lipid fraction accumulated in the liver in kwashiorkor is triglyceride. Thus the causes of fatty liver in kwashiorkor can be related to triglyceride metabolism. The most consistent finding in this respect is a very low level of plasma lipids, especially triglycerides (Schwartz and Dean, 112; Macdonald et al., 72; Lewis et al., 68; Flores et al., 33). It is also well documented that as soon as treatment starts there is a striking rise in serum lipids, again especially in serum triglycerides (Schwartz and Dean, 112; Macdonald et al., 72; Lewis et al., 68; Monckeberg, 78, 79; Flores et al., 33; Truswell and Hansen, 128; Truswell et al., 131). This rise during treatment led Schwartz and Dean to postulate that nutritional deficiencies in kwashiorkor would cause the lipids to be "locked" in the liver. This is at present the current hypothesis on the mechanism of fatty infiltration, as most of the data obtained in later work tend to provide support for it. A relative inability of the liver to dispose of triglycerides has been suggested as a contributory mechanism in almost all the hypotheses offered so far (Lewis et al., 68; Schendel and Hansen, 109; Fletcher, 32).

Waterlow (138) had identified protein as the dietary factor most likely to be responsible for the clearing of the liver fat during recovery. Lewis et al. (68) showed that the changes in serum lipids, especially in serum triglycerides, did not occur until protein was introduced in the diet. Feeding carbohydrate, however, produced a dramatic fall in the level of serum free fatty acids, which suggested that their high level is the result of the state of calorie deprivation of the patients, as the same authors pointed out.

The main metabolic pathway of liver triglycerides is their secretion into plasma in low-density lipoproteins. Cravioto et al. (28) and later Flores et al. (33) and Truswell et al. (130) have shown that the low-density lipoproteins are responsible both for the initial low level of serum lipids and their rise during recovery. This appears to be the main piece of evidence that supports the hypothesis of a block in the removal of liver triglycerides as the major factor in the pathogenesis of the fatty liver. In fact, fasting serum triglyceride levels are dependent on the synthesis of low-density lipoproteins solely by the liver (Byers and Friedman, 20; Harper et al., 45; Havel et al., 47; Havel and Goldfein, 46; Windmueller and Levy, 151). Thus the rise in the fasting levels of low-density lipoprotein-triglycerides during recovery would indicate defatting of the liver. The work in Chile (Flores et al., 33, 34) showed that coincident with these changes in serum lipids the liver lipid concentration fell to about 50% of the initial level within the first eight days of treatment (Fig. 1).

It is known from animal experiments that the synthesis of low-density lipoproteins can be inhibited, leading to fatty liver, by blocking the synthesis of any of the components of this lipoprotein, since experiments in rats (Heimberg et al., 53; Weinstein et al., 144) have shown that the components of the lipoprotein occur in constant proportions. Measurements on sera from patients recovering from kwashiorkor (Flores et al., 34) and from patients recovered from malnutrition, fed different diets (Seakins and Flores, 113) suggest that the observations in animals can be extrapolated to man. Figure 2 shows that the components of the serum $d < 1.019$ lipoprotein fraction do occur in a constant proportion in children. These measurements led to the further suggestion that in kwashiorkor the impairment lies at the level of the synthesis of the protein moiety of low-density lipoproteins. The argument has been based on the known low-protein intake in kwashiorkor and the markedly reduced levels of serum $\beta$-globulins (Monckeberg, 78, 79; Flores et al., 33, 34). This globulin fraction in all probability contains

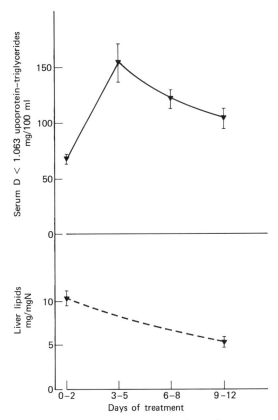

**Fig. 1.** The relationship between changes in triglyceride concentration in serum low-density lipoproteins and in liver lipids during treatment of kwashiorkor. (Taken from Flores et al., 34; with permission from the *British Journal of Nutrition*).

the circulating apoprotein of low-density lipoproteins described by Roheim et al. (102) and Lees (66). Truswell et al. (130) have also suggested an impairment in the synthesis of the apolipoprotein, based on the lack of evidence of a deficiency of lipotropic factors.

Experiments in rats have provided further support for this hypothesis. The administration of the serum protein fraction containing the lipo-protein-apoprotein to protein-depleted rats with fatty liver and low levels of fasting serum triglycerides caused a marked rise in the serum tri-glyceride concentration and increased incorporation of labeled oleic acid into serum low-density lipoprotein triglycerides (Flores et al., 34). These effects were not observed in normal rats, which suggests that in protein

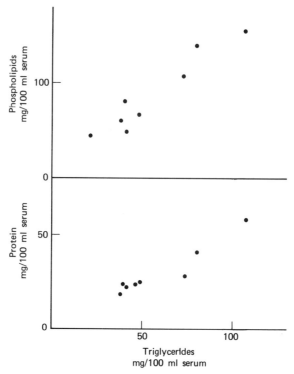

**Fig. 2.** Correlation between the concentration of components of human serum $d < 1.019$ lipoprotein. The lipoproteins were separated from the sera of patients with kwashiorkor on admission and during recovery as well as from recovered patients fed diets with varying proportions of fat. (Seakins and Flores, unpublished).

malnutrition the protein precursor of low-density lipoproteins becomes rate-limiting for their synthesis.

However, the generalization of the hypothesis reviewed above should be made with great care. Fatty livers can occur in kwashiorkor in the presence of high or normal levels of fasting serum triglycerides which fall steadily during recovery in some patients (Seakins and Flores, 113). In Jamaican children, who probably present the highest levels of liver lipids yet described (Waterlow, unpublished observations; Garrow et al., 37), the clearing of the liver fat is often a slow process (Waterlow, unpublished observations). Although a superimposed impairment in the removal of lipids from plasma could explain the observations in Jamaica, this is unlikely, since the adipose tissue is preserved in these patients as in those with kwashiorkor from other places (Garrow et al., 37).

By contrast they have elevated free fatty acid levels in plasma; this has been shown to be indicative of increased turnover (Lewis et al., 69).

The absence or infrequency of severe fatty infiltration in marasmus is still unexplained, since these patients have also received a protein-deficient diet. The major factor is presumably the low-calorie intake associated with marasmus. In addition, amino acids liberated by catabolism of tissue protein for energy may exert some protective effect. However unexplained, the differences between marasmus and kwashiorkor provide evidence that the disturbances of lipid metabolism studied so far are relevant to the pathogenesis of the fatty liver, since, except for the elevated level of serum free fatty acids, none of the changes reported in kwashiorkor are present in marasmus.

## PROTEIN METABOLISM

It is generally accepted that frank malnutrition in humans is found predominantly in infants and preschool children in the developing countries. Protein-calorie malnutrition (PCM) is a widely used term that describes a spectrum of disease embracing the three main clinical types—kwashiorkor, marasmus and marasmic-kwashiorkor. Their clinical features have been adequately described (Waterlow et al., 142). The actual worldwide incidence of PCM is not known nor is the incidence of subclinical or marginal malnutrition, which is estimated to be more prevalent, by several orders of magnitude, than frank PCM.

Intense international research in nutrition, in both practical and theoretical aspects, has been stimulated by this problem, which poses several questions of fundamental interest to medicine and physiology. The balance of mechanisms involved in human nutrition is at times subjected to additional stresses over and beyond the ordinary, and protein-calorie malnutrition in the young is a unique example of such a stress. Under these conditions survival may be equated to the ability of the body to adapt to prolonged dietary deficiencies of calories and protein.

In addition to the striking deficit in body weight, there are changes in the amount and distribution of protein, fat, minerals and water (Garrow et al., 37; Halliday, 44; Alleyne et al., 3). It seems most likely that these gross changes would be accompanied by and be related to adaptations in the normal homeostatic mechanisms that regulate the metabolism of body constituents, particularly of protein. Recent investigations have therefore been directed toward the elucidation of the dynamic aspects of protein metabolism in the protein-depleted child before, during, and after recovery from PCM.

One of the most consistent biochemical findings in kwashiorkor is a marked hypoalbuminaemia, and, with the development of isotope techniques it became possible to investigate the mechanisms leading to this phenomenon. Measurements have been made in the malnourished child of the distribution and rates of synthesis and catabolism of albumin to determine whether the hypoalbuminaemia of kwashiorkor was related to changes in the rates of synthesis or catabolism or to compartmental shifts of albumin or to a combination of these factors. Whatever the adaptive mechanisms, it was important to know if they resulted from the state of nutrition per se, the dietary intake of protein at the time of the test, or from both factors. The distribution and turnover of albumin were measured in the malnourished and recovered child by Gitlin and his coworkers in Mexico (1958) who injected [131]I-albumin intravenously into malnourished children and again after three to four weeks of treatment in hospital. They calculated the albumin half-life from the plasma decay curve of radioactivity, using Sterling's method (120); they found no change in the albumin half-life in malnutrition and concluded that in malnutrition the rate of catabolism of albumin was unaltered. It was subsequently pointed out that this conclusion was invalid (Waterlow et al., 142; Picou and Waterlow, 87; Cohen and Hansen, 26), since during the study on the malnourished children both plasma volume and plasma albumin concentration were increasing, which led to a dilution error and an apparent albumin half-life that was shorter than the true half-life. That difficulty was avoided by later workers who based their calculations of catabolic rate on the urinary excretion of labeled iodide, a method that is independent of steady-state conditions (Berson et al., 13; Cohen et al., 25). Picou and Waterlow (87) and Cohen and Hansen (26) showed that the albumin catabolic rate in the malnourished child was half that found after recovery. A causal relationship between nutritional state and catabolic rate of albumin was proposed by Picou and Waterlow (87), who stated that "the results reported here show that the nutritional state is a very important factor (influencing the breakdown of albumin) and it is tempting to suppose that the reduction in the rate of albumin breakdown in the malnourished children is a compensatory reaction to protein depletion." It was subsequently shown, however, that a fall in catabolic rate could be induced in normal adults after a week or more on a diet containing 10 g of protein a day, at which time the nutritional state of the subjects was only marginally affected (Hoffenberg et al., 55). On the evidence then available Waterlow (136) concluded that both dietary intake and nutritional state play a part in determining the rate of albumin catabolism. Because synthesis rates could not be measured directly in the studies cited above, no firm conclusions regarding the effects of protein depletion or protein intake on the rate of albumin synthesis could be drawn.

James and Hay (59) designed experiments to distinguish the effects of these two factors on albumin metabolism. A single dose of [131]I-albumin was administered and the level of dietary protein was altered after 7 to 10-day consecutive periods on a high- or low-protein intake. Both malnourished and recovered children were studied. The rate of synthesis of albumin was estimated by a computer analysis suitable for nonsteady-state conditions, and total activity of retained isotope was accurately measured during the month-long study by a whole body counter. The rates of synthesis and catabolism of albumin were calculated and the results are shown in Table 7. On a low-protein diet the synthesis rate

Table 7   The Effect of the Level of Protein Intake on the Absolute Rates of Synthesis and Catabolism of Albumin in Malnourished and Recovered Infants[a]

| Days of Study | 0–10 | 10–17 | 17–24[b] | 17–24[b] |
|---|---|---|---|---|
| Protein intake | High | Low | Low | High |
| Recovered children: | | | | |
| synthesis (mg albumin/kg-day) | 222 | 148 | 138 | 236 |
| catabolism (mg albumin/kg-day) | 219 | 178 | 140 | 156 |
| number of cases | 9 | 9 | 4 | 5 |
| Malnourished children: | | | | |
| synthesis (mg albumin/kg-day) | 233 | 101 | 87 | 288 |
| catabolism (mg albumin/kg-day) | 166 | 171 | 131 | 178 |
| Number of cases | 9 | 9 | 4 | 5 |

[a] Data from James and Hay (59). Reproduced by courtesy of the Editor of J.C.I.
[b] In the final dietary period (days 17–24) each group of nine children was divided into two subgroups: in one subgroup the low-protein diet was continued: in the other it was replaced by a high-protein intake.

in the malnourished children was significantly lower than that in the recovered children and was the same as that found by Cohen and Hansen (26) in their malnourished children. It rose when the level of dietary protein was increased and fell when it was lowered. These changes occurred promptly and were more marked in the malnourished children. Within a week of receiving a low-protein diet the absolute and fractional catabolic rates fell significantly in the recovered children, confirming similar results in adults (Hoffenberg et al., 55); a further fall occurred even when the protein intake was increased. In the malnourished children similar changes in the catabolic rate occurred when the protein content of the diet was altered. The delayed response of the catabolic rate to dietary alterations demonstrates that the protein intake does not directly control catabolic rate. This study also showed that changes in the catabolic rate were independent of albumin concentration and did not respond directly to changes in the synthesis rate.

In the above study the nonsteady-state condition brought about by dietary alterations necessitated the use of an indirect method to measure the rate of albumin synthesis. MacFarlane (73) introduced an independent and more direct method of measuring synthesis by using $^{14}C$-carbonate. This depends on comparing the total $^{14}C$ radioactivity incorporated into the guanidine carbon of albumin arginine with that incorporated into urea carbon in a given time, since both are synthesized from the same precursor. The method has been tested in the rat (Kirsch et al., 63) and in man (Tavill et al., 124) by comparing the rate of albumin synthesis, measured in this way, with the rate of catabolism measured simultaneously by the $^{131}I$-albumin method. Since the subjects were in a steady state, the two rates should be the same, as indeed they were. Kirsch et al. (63) found in rats on a protein-free diet that the synthesis rate promptly fell but that the decline in the catabolic rate occurred only after a definite time lag. On refeeding, there was an immediate increase in the synthesis rate, sometimes to higher than normal values, but a delayed rise in catabolic rate. The results were therefore in good agreement with those found in children by James and Hay (59).

The concept of compensatory or adaptive mechanisms of albumin metabolism to nutrient supply was first put forward by Hoffenberg (54, 55) and has been confirmed by subsequent workers. The picture that emerges from these investigations is that there is an immediate fall in albumin synthesis when the protein intake is reduced, and in order to maintain the intravascular albumin mass there is a net transfer of albumin from the extravascular to the intravascular pool. Later there is a compensatory decrease in catabolic rate, perhaps in response to a reduction in total albumin mass.

Further work has been concerned with how a change in dietary protein brings these adaptive mechanisms into play. Since the rate of albumin synthesis alters rapidly with changes in the level of dietary protein, it appears reasonable to postulate that the level or pattern of amino acids entering the liver may be an important factor controlling the rate of albumin synthesis. Rothschild et al. (103) measured the rate of albumin synthesis with $^{14}C$-carbonate, in the intact rabbit and the perfused liver when amino acids were either withheld or supplied. In studies on the whole animal there was a 33% decrease in albumin synthesis after an 18-to-24-hour fast and the perfused liver from fasted donors synthesized 53% less albumin than a similar preparation from a fed donor. In a later study Rothschild et al. (104) reported that albumin synthesis by the livers from fasted rabbits increased by 89% when isoleucine (10 $\mu$m/ml) and by 138% when tryptophan (.05 $\mu$m/ml) were added to the perfusate. Other amino acids, either singly or in combination, did not alter the amount of albumin synthesized when added to the perfusate. Kirsch et al. (64) used a different approach and perfused isolated livers from well-fed rats with blood from donor rats fed a low-protein diet for two days. This donor blood contained low levels of the branched chain amino acids, and the perfused liver synthesized significantly less albumin than when it was perfused with blood from fed donor rats. A normal rate of albumin synthesis was achieved when the perfusate blood from starved donor rats was supplemented with branched chain amino acids to restore the normal amino acid pattern. It is interesting to note that in malnourished infants and in normal subjects receiving a low-protein diet albumin synthesis is decreased and the branched chain essential amino acids are reduced in plasma. However, the relationship between albumin synthetic activity in the liver and the level or pattern of amino acids it receives is clearly more complex than the apparently straightforward results of these studies. Not only may the levels of intracellular and plasma free amino acids differ but the intracellular free amino acids may be selectively distributed to microsomes, nuclei, mitochondria, or other morphological sites at which protein synthesis is known to occur. Clarification of the role of the level and pattern of plasma amino acids in albumin metabolism awaits further study, but it is pertinent to consider some aspects of amino acid metabolism in overall protein malnutrition.

In malnourished children the total amount of plasma amino acids is reduced to about one-half the normal value (Arroyave, 7), and a distorted pattern has been reported in patients with kwashiorkor from several parts of the world (Holt et al., 56). There is reduction in the levels of several essential amino acids plus tyrosine with little change or some elevation in the levels of the nonessential amino acids. Whitehead (149) introduced a semiquantitative method to measure the degree of distortion of the plasma aminogram by expressing as a ratio (the N/E ratio) a selected number of nonessential and essential amino acids. The ratio was found to be high (greater than 2) in patients with kwashiorkor in Uganda but was not raised in marasmus, and it was claimed that an elevated N/E ratio was indicative of protein deficiency

(Whitehead, 150). Subsequently, workers in other parts of the world reported results that supported this hypothesis (Arroyave and Bowering, 8). It is questionable, however whether the distorted plasma aminogram reflects solely the state of protein nutrition of the individual. Saunders et al. (108) showed that in kwashiorkor the altered plasma amino acid pattern reverted to normal after only one day of treatment. Similarly in five children with kwashiorkor the initially high N/E ratio fell to normal values after two to three weeks of treatment, long before clinical recovery had been achieved (Arroyave and Bowering, 8). Also, workers in the Lebanon and South Africa have failed to demonstrate a raised N/E ratio in severe kwashiorkor (McLaren et al., 74; Truswell et al., 131). A distorted plasma aminogram, like that found in kwashiorkor, or a high N/E ratio can be produced in healthy adults after a short period (1 to 15 days) on a low-protein diet and before any significant loss of body protein occurs (Swendseid et al., 123; Young and Scrimshaw, 158; Weller et al., 145). Finally, Holt (56) has reported that premature infants who were growing normally developed a plasma aminogram similar to that found in kwashiorkor.

It is clear that there is no single factor responsible for the altered amino acid pattern after fasting or in protein-deficient states, and an investigation into the possible mechanisms responsible for the altered levels of plasma amino acids might lead to a better understanding of their role in regulating synthesis and catabolism of protein. Amino acids arise from exogenous and endogenous sources, and the pattern in the extracellular pool, represented by the plasma aminogram, reflects the balance between supply from these sources and the demands imposed by maintenance and growth (protein synthesis), catabolism mainly to urea, and energy requirements. The interplay of these reactions among the several amino acids produces a complex picture in which it is difficult to discern cause and effect. By varying one factor, the level of dietary protein, and observing how the plasma aminogram alters it may be possible to infer what mechanisms are likely to have been involved. Arroyave et al. (8) reduced the protein intake of children in a stepwise fashion and found that the N/E ratio began to rise when the protein intake fell below 1 g/kg, which is slightly less than the value proposed by the WHO/FAO (1965) as the requirement of children aged 1 year.* In a similar experiment with young pigs it was found that the N/E ratio became elevated when the dietary intake ceased to support growth. It was postulated that up to that time the amino acid supply

* WHO, *Tech. Rep. Series No. 301.* Report of a joint FAO/WHO Expert Group (1965).

was in excess of or equal to the demand, but that beyond that period reduced levels of amino acids would be expected. Although this may explain a general reduction in amino acid levels, it does not explain why certain branched chain essential amino acids are preferentially decreased in the plasma. The latter finding may be explained by the observation that the activity of branched chain amino acid transaminases is much higher in muscle and kidney than in liver and that enzyme activity in muscle is doubled when a low protein diet is fed to rats. In contrast to this possibility of enhanced catabolism of branched chain amino acids leading to a reduction in their plasma levels, the relatively normal levels of histidine, phenylalanine, and lysine could be due to their abnormal catabolism (Holt et al., 56; Whitehead and Dean, 149; Whitehead, 146) in kwashiorkor.

Of the nonessential amino acids, alanine appears not to be significantly altered in the plasma of malnourished children. This is in contrast to the finding in adults of a marked fall in plasma alanine during the first few days of starvation (Felig et al., 31) and a significant rise after one day on a protein-free diet (Weller et al., 145). Felig et al. (31) have postulated that in starvation there is an increased and preferential hepatic utilization of alanine for gluconeogenesis (alanine being one of the key amino acids in gluconeogenesis) so that glucose is supplied to the brain until that organ becomes adapted to keto-acid utilization.

At present it appears that some of the factors contributing to a distorted plasma aminogram in protein malnutrition include an altered metabolism in muscle, enhanced liver gluconeogenesis, and abnormal metabolism of certain amino acids. The levels of amino acids by themselves, however, tell us little of the rates of uptake of amino acids into protein, and a more fruitful approach is to study the dynamic aspects of amino acid and protein metabolism.

The adaptation of albumin metabolism in response to alteration in the diet or nutritional state does not necessarily represent the metabolic behavior of other body proteins. This becomes apparent in the following review of total protein metabolism in man. Although suitable isotopic techniques and methodology have enabled the kinetics of albumin metabolism in man to be defined fairly accurately, measurements of the overall rates of protein synthesis and catabolism in man have been relatively few and, because of the complex nature of the problem, are deliberately based on oversimplified models of protein metabolism. The concept of total nitrogen or protein turnover is inherent in the view of the living cell as a dynamic system (Schoenheimer, 111), and Rechgigl (100) has cogently marshaled the available evidence in support of this concept. It is by regulation of protein turnover and of rates of synthesis and catabolism of protein that the body adapts to alterations in the level of dietary intake. Waterlow has illustrated this point in his discussion of the possible ways these mechanisms may operate to bring about one of the fundamental adaptations in protein metabolism, namely, the fall in urinary nitrogen that occurs when protein intake is reduced.

Total nitrogen turnover may be defined as the amount of amino nitrogen, derived from food and from catabolism of tissue proteins, that enters a metabolic pool in a given period of time or leaves it by synthesis into protein or excretion in the urine. It represents the sum of all the turnovers in all the individual tissues and of all the proteins in those tissues. It is therefore an entity of the same kind as the basal metabolic rate which is the sum of the rates of oxygen turnover in all the cells of the body. The overall rate of protein synthesis in man has been estimated under normal conditions (Sprinson and Rittenberg, 117; Wu and Snyderman, 152; San Pietro and Rittenberg, 107; Olesen et al., 85), in diseased states (Crispell et al., 29; Torizuka et al., 125), and in different nutritional states (Tschudy et al., 132). Most of these measurements were made after a single injection of a labeled isotope, usually [15]N-glycine; calculations of the rate of synthesis have been based on three main methods: (a) the time taken for maximum isotope enrichment to be reached in urinary urea (San Pietro and Rittenberg, 107), (b) measurement of pool size and turnover rate of a single amino acid from the plasma decay curve of the injected labeled amino acid, and (c) the cumulative excretion or retention of isotope over several days after a single injection of the labeled amino acid. There are valid grounds for criticizing all these methods (Wu and Bishop, 153; Tschudy et al., 132; Wu et al., 155). Waterlow and Stephen (140), who have summarized these criticisms, devised a constant infusion method to study the kinetics of protein metabolisms after preliminary work with [35]S-methionine (Picou and Waterlow, 88). If a labeled amino acid is given, the rate at which it is synthesized into protein can be calculated if the specific activity of the immediate precursor, i.e., the tracer amino acid at the site of synthesis, and of the product are measured simultaneously. However, when a single dose of labeled amino acid is given, its specific activity changes rapidly and in a complex manner with time. Because of this, accurate serial measurements of specific activities of precursor and product present great difficulties. If, however, the labeled amino acid is continuously infused, the specific activity of the given amino acid will rise to a plateau, provided that reentry of label is insignificant (Zilversmit, 159). After continuous intravenous infusions of [14]C-lysine in rats (Waterlow and Stephen, 140, 141) and in man (Waterlow, 137) the specific activity of the labeled amino acid reached a

plateau in the plasma. The findings of Gan and Jeffay (36) who infused
[14]C-phenylalanine in rats confirmed those obtained by Waterlow. On
the basis of these experiments Picou and Taylor-Roberts (89) devised
a constant-infusion method using [15]N-glycine to measure the overall
rates of nitrogen turnover and synthesis and catabolism of protein in
infants. They investigated the effects of nutritional state and dietary
intake on these rates. The constant-infusion method and its assumptions
are examined in some detail, since the results obtained indicate quantitatively some of the adaptive responses in man to alterations in nutritional state and dietary intake of protein.

The model used (Fig. 3) depicts in a simplified form the kinetic
relationship between amino acid and protein metabolism that is known

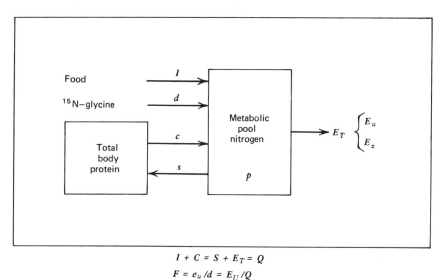

$$I + C = S + E_T = Q$$
$$F = e_u/d = E_U/Q$$
$$Q = E_U/F$$

Fig. 3. Schematic diagram of the [15]N-glycine constant infusion method (Picou and
Taylor-Roberts, 89).

to occur in man. It offers the advantage that some of its assumptions
can be experimentally tested; also, mathematical treatment of the data
is simple, since the method of constant infusion achieves an isotopic
steady state. Amino acids from the diet and from catabolism of body
protein enter a metabolic pool $P$ and are either synthesized into protein
or degraded and excreted in the urine as nitrogenous products, mainly
as urea. $I$, $C$, $S$, and $E_T$ denote, respectively, the rates (milligrams N

per hour) of entry of amino N from the diet and from tissue catabolism, the rate of synthesis into protein, and the rate of excretion of total N in urine. $E_T$ is the sum of $E_U$, the rate of excretion of urinary urea N, and $E_X$, the rate of excretion of nonurea N (milligrams per hour). [15]N-glycine is infused at the rate of $d$ mg [15]N/hr. In an isotopic steady state the proportion $F$ of infused [15]N excreted as labeled urea is the same as the proportion of the total amino N entering the pool excreted as urea. This can be expressed as:

$$F = \frac{e}{d} = \frac{E_U}{Q} \tag{1}$$

where, in time $t$, $e$ is the amount of [15]N excreted as urea, which can be measured, and $Q$ is the N turnover or the amount of amino N entering the pool; since $F$ and $E_U$ are known, $Q$ can be calculated. If the size of the metabolic pool $P$ remains constant during the period when measurements are made, then

$$Q = I + C = E + S \tag{2}$$

and $S$ and $C$, the rates of synthesis and catabolism, respectively, can be calculated from (2). The size of the metabolic pool $P$ cannot be measured by this method, and the assumption that it was constant during the period that measurements were taken could not be tested. Nor was it possible to test whether reentry of isotope was significant during the experiment. The authors point out, however, that since the enrichment of urinary urea was constant during the latter part of the infusion (plateau period) it was unlikely that isotope reentry was significant or that the size of the metabolic pool was inconstant during the plateau period.

It was important to determine whether the body handles amino acids derived from food and from tissue breakdown in a like manner, since for practical reasons the intragastric route is preferable to the intravenous route for continuous infusions. There is the possibility that amino acids which are absorbed from the gastrointestinal tract and transported to the liver may be catabolized to urea more readily than amino acids derived from tissue catabolism. This point was tested by comparing the N turnover rates obtained by consecutive intragastric and intravenous infusions in the same infant under the same conditions. In two infants the turnover rates obtained by infusing the isotope by the two routes were in close agreement. It can therefore be accepted that for practical purposes amino acids of exogenous and endogenous origins may be considered as mixing in a homogenous metabolic pool. Another important point to be tested was whether the urinary data reflected the metabolic fate of the administered amino acid or of the amino acid pool as a whole. From results of experiments in which a [15]N-amino acid was given as a single oral dose Wu and his colleagues concluded that in the first few hours urinary data reflected the metabolism of the administered amino acid (Wu and Bishop, 153; Wu and Sendroy, 154; Wu et al., 155). To test this point Picou and Taylor-Roberts (89) compared the results obtained from consecutive intragastric infusions of [15]N-glycine and [15]N-labeled egg protein in the same child under identical conditions. In two infants the rates of synthesis, catabolism, and N turnover after infusing the two labeled substances were the same. It is therefore clear that [15]N-glycine is a valid tracer of the amino acid pool when used in the constant-infusion method.

The effects of malnutrition on the rates of synthesis and catabolism and N turnover were investigated by measuring these rates in five children when they were malnourished and again when they had completely recovered some six weeks later. The protein intake, 3.5 g/kg, was kept the same in the two studies. The results are shown in Table 8. In recovered

**Table 8   Mean Values for Nitrogen Turnover ($Q$), Synthesis ($S$) and Catabolism ($C$) of Total Body Protein in Five Infants before and after Recovery from Malnutrition**

|  | Malnourished | Recovered | $p$ |
|---|---|---|---|
| $Q$ mg N/kg-hr | 88 | 56 | $< .05$ |
| $S$ g protein/kg-day | 11.2 | 6.1 | $< .025$ |
| $C$ g protein/kg-day | 9.7 | 4.7 | $< .0125$ |

children the rate of total protein synthesis was twice that found in normal adults (unpublished data) and significantly higher than that reported by Wu and Snyderman (152) for normal infants. The malnourished children had strikingly higher rates of synthesis and catabolism and N turnover than when they had recovered. Although net protein synthesis was the same in the two studies, the malnourished children were more efficient in utilizing available N for synthesis than when they had recovered (see Table 9). It is tempting to speculate on the mechanisms that may be responsible for this hypermetabolic state in malnutrition. Alleyne and Young (2) have shown that in malnourished infants, similar to those studied by Picou and Taylor-Roberts (89),

Table 9   Percentage of the N Entering the Pool Synthesized into Protein ($S/Q \times 100$) and Derived from Catabolism of Protein ($C/Q \times 100$) in Five Infants before and after Recovery from Malnutrition[a]

| | $S/Q \times 100$ | | $C/Q \times 100$ | |
|---|---|---|---|---|
| Subject | Malnourished | Recovered | Malnourished | Recovered |
| Del B. | 79 | 76 | 69 | 54 |
| Der B. | 73 | 67 | 66 | 44 |
| D.C. | 88 | 74 | 71 | 69 |
| J.D. | 93 | 74 | 82 | 54 |
| L.L. | 93 | 70 | 79 | 66 |
| Mean | 85 | 73 | 73 | 57 |
| $p$ | $< .01$ | | $< .01$ | |

[a] Measurements made at equal levels of protein intake.

plasma cortisol levels were high. Also in malnutrition plasma insulin was low and glucose stimulation provoked little or no rise in insulin level (James and Coore, 60). The catabolic effect of cortisol on carcass protein is well documented (see Munro, 81) and the high levels in the malnourished child could partly explain the increase in protein catabolism. It is also possible that since physiological increases in the level of circulating insulin inhibit net release of amino acids from muscle (Posefsky et al., 94) the reverse effect could occur so that the low insulin levels in the malnourished child may enhance the output of amino acids from muscle. Plasma-growth hormone level is also raised in protein malnutrition (Pimstone et al., 90, 91, 92; Milner, 77) and may well be related to the increased rate of protein synthesis in the malnourished child.

The effect of protein intake on overall protein metabolism was investigated by Picou and Taylor-Roberts (89), who measured synthetic and catabolic rates of protein and N turnover in well-nourished children who were fed isocaloric high- and low-protein diets for consecutive periods. The results are shown in Table 10. On a low-protein diet containing 1.2 g of protein per kilogram per day the net retention of N was low, and this is to be expected, since the protein intake was just sufficient to allow the infant to grow at a slow rate. However, the absolute rate of protein synthesis was the same on the two diets and there was a more efficient utilization of amino N when the protein intake was low (Table 11). When protein intake is lowered, it seems that catabolism

Table 10    Mean Values for Nitrogen Turnover $(Q)$, Synthesis $(S)$ and Catabolism $(C)$ of Total Body Protein in Six Recovered Infants on a High- and a Low-Protein Intake

|  | Low Protein | High Protein | $p$ |
|---|---|---|---|
| $Q$ mg N/kg-hr | 45 | 62 | $< .0025$ |
| $S$ g protein/kg-day | 6.2 | 6.5 | N.S. |
| $C$ g protein/kg-day | 5.5 | 4.2 | $< .05$ |

Table 11    Percentage of N Entering the Pool Synthesized into Protein $(S/Q \times 100)$ and Derived from Catabolism of Protein $(C/Q \times 100)$ in Recovered Infants on a Low- and a High-Protein Intake

| Subject | $S/Q \times 100$ | | $C/Q \times 100$ | |
|---|---|---|---|---|
|  | Low Protein | High Protein | Low Protein | High Protein |
| Del B. | 94 | 76 | 83 | 54 |
|  |  | 69 |  | 29 |
| Der B. | 92 | 67 | 82 | 44 |
|  |  | 65 |  | 42 |
| D.C. | 94 | 71 | 85 | 48 |
| W.W. | 91 | — | 77 | — |
| V.T. | 91 | — | 82 | — |
| S.C. | — | 67 | — | 48 |
| Mean | 92 | 69 | 82 | 44 |

accounts for about 80% of the amino acids entering the metabolic pool. Of this flux of amino acids 90% is synthesized into protein and very little is lost as urea. It is with these mechanisms that the body adapts to a lowered protein intake. This preferential pathway of amino acids to protein synthesis rather than to urea formation was also demonstrated by the malnourished child. It has been shown in rats that a low-protein diet causes a decrease in the total liver content of urea cycle enzymes (Schimke, 110) and an increase in the activity of amino acid activating enzymes (Mariani et al., 75). Stephen and Waterlow (119) showed similar changes in enzyme activity in the livers of infants studied before and after recovery from malnutrition. The more efficient utilization of amino acids for protein synthesis in both the malnourished infant and the normal infant receiving a low-protein diet may be brought about by these enzyme changes which we believe to be adaptive.

It has long been known that urea, far from being a metabolically inert end product of protein catabolism, undergoes further metabolic changes in the body. Schoenheimer (111) and Bloch (15) found that labeled protein and ammonia appeared in the carcass of rats after $^{15}$N-urea was administered and Walser and Bodelos (134) calculated that about 15 to 30% of urea synthesized did not appear as urinary urea and presumably underwent further metabolic transformation. Regoeczi et al. (101) calculated that in rabbits less than half of the urea produced was excreted in the urine. These observations lead us to ask what the role of urea N is in overall N metabolism. Before urea can be utilized in the body, it is first hydrolysed to $NH_3$ by bacterial ureases in the gastrointestinal tract (Chao and Tarver, 23; Levenson et al., 67). The $NH_3$ so produced may be resynthesized into urea or enter into pathways leading to protein synthesis.

Regoeczi et al. (101) injected $^{14}$C-urea and $^{15}$N-urea simultaneously in rabbits and calculated from the slopes of the disappearance in plasma of the two isotopes that of the $^{15}$N-urea present in plasma 21% was due to recyclying of the isotope. Jones et al. (62) consider that in normal adults on an adequate protein intake this enterohepatic circulation of the N of urea, amounting to some 2 to 4 g N/day, constitutes a delay pathway in the excretion of N.

From the available evidence it seems quite clear that the N resulting from deamination of urea by intestinal bacteria can be synthesized into urea. There is equally convincing evidence that it may also be synthesized into protein. Normal infants who had ceased to grow when on an inadequate protein intake resumed normal growth when urea was added to the diet, and when $^{15}$N urea was given the label was found in plasma protein and haemoglobin, showing the urea-N was used for protein synthesis (Snyderman et al., 116). During the 48 hours after an intravenous dose of $^{15}$N-urea in three marasmic infants retentions of 16 to 31% of the administered $^{15}$N were found, compared with only 1 and 11% in two controls (Read et al., 99). These authors also calculated that less urea was resynthesized and more urea was metabolized in marasmic than in normal infants.

Although these and other studies (see Read et al., 99) indicate that the N of urea or $NH_3$ is recycled as well as incorporated into protein, there are no measurements of the relative amounts involved in the two processes. Synthesis of nonessential N into protein occurs to a greater extent when the diet is inadequate in nitrogen and when the subject is malnourished. It is quite probable that in normal subjects on an adequate diet urea is involved to a significant extent in the N economy of the body. Interruption of the enterohepatic pathway may lead to a negative N balance. It is reasonable to postulate that supplementing a diet with nonessential N would lead to positive N balance only if the limiting factor in the diet is "unessential nitrogen." It is difficult, however, to envisage how, in the absence of an adequate supply of essential amino acids or their carbon skeletons, urea N, $NH_3$, or any other form of nonessential N can contribute to net protein synthesis.

## REFERENCES

1. S. A. Adibi, *Amer. J. Physiol.* **25**: 52 (1968).
2. G. A. O. Alleyne and V. H. Young, *Clin. Sci.* **33**: 189 (1967).
3. G. A. O. Alleyne and G. H. Scullard, *Clin. Sci.* **37**: 631 (1969).
4. G. A. O. Alleyne and G. H. Scullard, *Amer. J. Clin. Nutr.* **22**: 1139 (1969).
5. G. A. O. Alleyne, D. Halliday, J. C. Waterlow, and B. L. Nichols, *Brit. J. Nutr.* **23**: 783 (1969).
6. G. A. O. Alleyne and H. S. Besterman, Paper submitted.
7. G. Arroyave, D. Wilson, C. De Funes, and M. Behar, *Amer. J. Clin. Nutr.* **11**: 517 (1962).
8. G. Arroyave and J. Bowering, *Arch. Latinoam. Nutr.* **18**: 341 (1968).
9. H. A. Baig, and J. C. Edozien, *Lancet* **ii**: 662 (1965).
10. R. W. R. Baker and I. MacDonald, *Nature* **189**: 406 (1961).
11. J. M. Bengoa, *Proc. 8th Intern. Congr. Nutr.*, Prague (1969).
12. J. Bergstrom and E. Hultman, *Nature* **210**: 309 (1966).
13. S. A. Berson, R. S. Yalow, S. S. Schreiber, and J. Post, *J. Clin. Invest.* **32**: 746 (1953).
14. H. S. Besterman, and G. A. O. Alleyne, In press.
15. K. Bloch, *J. Biol. Chem.* **165**: 469 (1946).
16. M. D. Bowie, *S. Afr. Med. J.* **38**: 328 (1964).
17. M. D. Bowie, G. O. Barbezat, and J. D. L. Hansen, *Amer. J. Clin. Nutr.* **20**: 89 (1967).
18. B. Bronte-Stewart, in *Recent Advances in Human Nutrition.* J. F. Brock, Ed. London: Churchill, 1961.
19. R. M. Buckle, *Clin. Sci.* **31**: 181 (1966).
20. S. O. Byers and M. Friedman, *Amer. J. Physiol.* **198**: 629 (1960).
21. J. P. Carter, A. Kaatab, K. Abd-el-Hadi, J. T. Davis, A. El Gholmy, and V. N. Patwardhan, *Amer. J. Clin. Nutr.* **21**: 195 (1968).
22. H. Chan and J. C. Waterlow, *Brit. J. Nutr.* **20**: 755 (1966).
23. F. C. Chao and H. Tarver, *Proc. Soc. Expt. Biol. N.Y.* **84**: 406 (1953).
24. K. K. Chatterjee and K. L. Mukherjee, *Brit. J. Nutr.* **22**: 145 (1968).
25. S. Cohen, T. Freeman, and A. S. McFarlane, *Clin. Sic.* **20**: 161 (1961).

26. S. Cohen and J. D. L. Hansen, *Clin. Sci.* **23**: 351 (1962).

27. G. C. Cook, *Nature* **215**: 1295 (1967).

28. J. Cravioto, C. L. De la Pena, and G. Burgos, *Metabolism* **8**: 722 (1959).

29. K. R. Crispell, W. Parson, and G. Hollifield. *J. Clin. Invest.* **35**: 164 (1956).

30. R. F. A. Dean, *Mod. Probl. Paediat.* **2**: 133 (1957).

31. P. Felig, O. E. Owen, J. Wahren, and G. F. Cahill, *J. Clin. Invest.* **48**: 584 (1969).

32. K. Fletcher, *Amer. J. Clin. Nutr.* **15**: 161 (1966).

33. H. Flores, N. Pak, A. Maccioni, and F. Monckeberg, *Abstracts 37th Ann. Meeting Soc. Pediat. Res., 1967*, Atlantic City, New Jersey (1967).

34. H. Flores, W. Sierralta, and F. Monckeberg, *J. Nutr.* **106**: 375 (1970).

35. H. Flores, N. Pak, A. Maccioni, and F. Monckeberg, *Brit. J. Nutr.* **24**: 1005 (1970).

36. J. C. Gan and H. Jeffay, *Biochim. Biophys. Acta* **148**: 448 (1967).

37. J. S. Garrow, K. Fletcher, and D. Halliday, *J. Clin. Invest.* **44**: 417 (1965).

38. J. S. Garrow, *Arch. Latinoam. Nutr.* **26**: 145 (1966).

39. J. Gillman, T. Gillman, J. Scragg, N. Savage, C. Gilbert, G. Trout, and P. Levy, *S. Afr. J. Med. Sci.* **26**: 31 (1961).

40. D. Gitlin, J. Cravioto, S. Frenk, E. L. Montano, R. Ramos-Galvan, F. Gomez, and C. A. Janeway, *J. Clin. Invest.* **37**: 682 (1958).

41. F. Gomez, R. Ramos-Galvan, S. Frenk, J. M. Cravioto, R. Chavez, and J. Vazquez, *J. Trop. Pediat.* **2**: 77 (1956).

42. G. G. Graham, A. Cordano, and R. M. Blizzard, *Paed. Res.* **3**: 579 (1969).

43. D. R. Hadden, *Lancet* **ii**: 589 (1967).

44. D. Halliday, *Clin. Sci.* **33**: 365 (1967).

45. P. V. Harper, Jr., W. B. Neal, Jr. and G. R. Hlavacek, *Metabolism* **2**: 62 (1953).

46. R. J. Havel and A. Goldfier, *J. Lipid. Res.* **2**: 389 (1961).

47. R. J. Havel, J. M. Felts, and C. M. Jan Duyne, *J. Lipid Res.* **3**: 297 (1962).

48. C. R. C. Heard, *Diabetes* **15**: 78 (1966).

49. C. R. C. Heard and M. R. Turner, *Diabetes* **16**: 96 (1967).

50. C. R. C. Heard, P. A. J. Henry, M. Hartog, and A. D. Wright, *Proc. Nutr. Soc.* **27**: 6A (1968).

51. C. R. C. Heard, and P. A. J. Henry, *J. Endocrin.* **45**: 375–386 (1969).

52. C. R. C. Heard, and P. A. J. Henry, *Clin. Sci.* **37**: 37 (1969).

53. M. Heimberg, I. Weinstein, G. Dishmon, and M. Fried, *Amer. J. Physiol.* **209**: 1053 (1965).

54. R. Hoffenberg, S. Saunders, G. C. Linder, E. Black, and J. F. Brock, in *Protein Metabolism*, F. Gross, Ed. Berlin: Springer, 1962, p. 314.

55. R. Hoffenberg, E. Black, and J. F. Brock, *J. Clin. Invest.* **45**: 143 (1966).

56. L. E. Holt, S. E. Snyderman, P. M. Norton, E. Roitman, and J. Finch, *Lancet* **ii**: 1343 (1963).

57. L. L. Hopkins, O. Ransome-Kuti, and A. S. Majaj, *Amer. J. Clin. Nutr.* **21**: 203 (1968).

58. W. P. T. James, *Lancet* **i**: 333 (1968).

58A. W. P. T. James, *Clin. Sci.* 39: 305 (1970).

59. W. P. T. James and A. M. Hay, *J. Clin. Invest.* 47: 1958 (1968).

60. W. P. T. James, and H. G. Coore, *Amer. J. Clin. Nutr.* 23: 386 (1970).

61. E. A. Jones, A. Craigie, A. S. Tavill, W. Simon, and V. M. Rosenoer, *Clin. Sci.* 35: 553 (1968).

62. E. A. Jones, R. A. Smallwood, Anne Craigie, and V. M. Rosenoer, *Clin. Sci.* 37: 825 (1969).

63. R. Kirsch, L. Frith, E. Black, and R. Hoffenberg, *Nature* 217: 578 (1968).

64. R. E. Kirsch, S. J. Saunders, L. Frith, S. Wight, and J. F. Brock, *S. Afr. Med. J.* 43: 125 (1969).

65. R. E. Kirsch, S. J. Saunders, L. Frith, S. Wicht, L. Kelman, and J. F. Brock, *Amer. J. Clin. Nutr.* 22: 1559 (1969).

66. Robert L. Lees, *J. Lipid Res.* 8: 396 (1967).

67. S. M. Levenson, L. V. Crowley, R. E. Horowitz, and O. J. Malm, *J. Biol. Chem.* 234: 2061 (1959).

68. B. Lewis, J. D. L. Hansen, W. Wittman, L. H. Krut, and F. Stewart, *Amer. J. Clin. Nutr.* 15: 161 (1964).

69. B. Lewis, W. Wittman, L. H. Krut, J. D. L. Hansen, and J. F. Brock, *Clin. Sci.* 30: 371 (1966).

70. I. MacDonald, *Metabolism* 9: 838 (1960).

71. I. MacDonald, *Amer. J. Clin. Nutr.* 10: 111 (1962).

72. I. MacDonald, J. D. L. Hansen, and B. Bronte-Stewart, *Clin. Sci.* 24: 55 (1963).

73. A. S. McFarlane, *Biochem. J.* 87: 22P (1963).

74. D. S. McLaren, W. W. Kamel, and N. Ayyoub, *Amer. J. Clin. Nutr.* 17: 152 (1965).

75. A. Mariani, P. A. Migliaccio, M. A. Spadoni, and M. Ticca, *J. Nutr.* 90: 25 (1966).

76. J. Metcoff, S. Frenk, T. Yoshida, R. Torees Pinedo, E. Kaiser, and J. D. L. Hansen, *Medicine* 45: 365 (1966).

77. R. D. G. Milner, *Malnutrition and the Endocrine System in Man*, Men. Soc. Endocrinol. 18: 191 (1970).

78. F. Monckeberg, *Nutr. Bromatol. Toxicol.* 5: 31 (1966).

79. F. Monckeberg, in *Calorie Deficiencies and Protein Deficiencies*, R. A. McCance and E. M. Widdowson. Eds. London: Churchill, 1968.

80. K. L. Mukherjee and R. L. Noth, *Bull. Calcutta Soc. Trop. Med.* 5: 170 (1957).

81. H. Munro, in *Mammalian Protein Metabolism*, J. Allison and H. Munro, Eds. New York: Academic, 1964.

82. W. E. Nelson, *Textbook of Pediatrics*, 7th ed. Philadelphia: Saunders, 1959.

83. B. L. Nichols, C. F. Hazelwood, and D. J. Branes, *J. Pediat.* 72: 840 (1968).

84. B. L. Nichols, C. F. Hazlewood, J. Alvarado, and F. Viteri, *Fed. Proc.* 28: 807 (1969).

85. K. Oleson, N. C. S. Heilskov, and F. Schonheyder, *Biochim. Biophys. Acta.* 15: 95 (1954).

86. S. Oxman, A. Maccioni, A. Zuniga, R. Spada, and F. Monckeberg, *Amer. J. Clin. Nutr.* **21:** 1285 (1968).

87. D. Picou and J. C. Waterlow, *Clin. Sci.* **22:** 459 (1962).

88. D. Picou, and J. C. Waterlow, in *Amino Acid Metabolism and Genetic variation.* W. L. Nyhan, Ed. New York: McGraw-Hill, 1967, p. 421.

89. D. Picou, and T. Taylor-Roberts, *Clin. Sci.* **36:** 283 (1969).

90. B. L. Pimstone, W. Wittman, J. D. L. Hansen, and P. Murray, *Lancet* **ii:** 779 (1966).

91. B. L. Pimstone, G. Barbezat, J. D. L. Hansen, and P. Murray, *Lancet* **ii:** 1333 (1967).

92. B. L. Pimstone, G. Barbezat, J. D. L. Hansen, and P. Murray, *Amer. J. Clin. Nutr.* **21:** 482 (1968).

93. B. S. Platt, K. Halder, and B. H. Doell, *Proc. Nutr. Soc.* **21:** vi (1962).

94. T. Posefsky, P. Felig, J. D. Tobin, J. S. Soeldner, and G. F. Cahill, *J. Clin. Invest.* **48:** 2273 (1969).

95. K. S. J. Rao, *Amer. J. Dis. Child.* **110:** 519 (1965).

96. K. S. J. Rao, *Ind. J. Biochem.* **2:** 183 (1965).

97. K. S. J. Rao and P. S. K. Prasad, *Amer. J. Clin. Nutr.* **19:** 205 (1966).

98. K. S. J. Rao, S. G. Srikantia, and C. Gopalan, *Arch. Dis. Child.* **43:** 365 (1968).

99. W. W. C. Read, D. S. McLaren, M. Tchalian, and S. Nassar, *J. Clin. Invest.* **48:** 1143 (1969).

100. M. Recheigl, *Tex. Rep. Biol. Med.* **26:** 147 (1968).

101. F. Regoeczi, L. Irons, A. Koj, and A. S. McFarlane, *Biochem. J.* **95:** 521 (1965).

102. P. S. Roheim, L. Miller, and H. A. Eder, *J. Biol. Chem.* **240:** 2994 (1965).

103. M. Rothschild, M. Oratz, J. Mongelli, and S. S. Schreiber, *J. Clin. Invest.* **47:** 2591 (1968).

104. M. A. Rothschild, M. Oratz, J. Mongelli, L. Fishman, and S. S. Schreiber, *J. Nutr.* **98:** 395 (1969).

105. I. H. E. Rutishauser and R. G. Whitehead, *Brit. J. Nutr.* **23:** 1 (1969).

106. C. Salazar de Sousa, *Pediatria int.* (*Roma*) **9:** 167 (1959).

107. A. San Pietro and D. Rittenberg, *J. Biol. Chem.* **201:** 457 (1953).

108. S. J. Saunders, A. S. Truswell, G. O. Barbezat, W. Wittman, and J. D. L. Hansen, *Lancet* **ii:** 795 (1967).

109. H. E. Schendal, and J. D. L. Hansen, *Amer. J. Clin. Nutr.* **9:** 735 (1961).

110. R. T. Schimke, *J. Biol. Chem.* **237:** 1921 (1962).

111. R. Schoenheimer, in *The Dynamic State of Body Constituents.* Cambridge, Mass.: Harvard University Press, 1942.

112. R. Schwartz, and R. F. A. Dean, *J. Trop. Pediat.* **3:** 23 (1957).

113. A. Seakins and H. Flores, *15th Sci Meeting of SACMR*, UWI, Jamaica (1970).

114. E. Shrago and H. A. Lardy, *J. Biol. Chem.* **241:** 663 (1966).

115. D. Sloane, L. S. Tait, and G. S. Gilchrist, *Brit. Med. J.* **i:** 32 (1961).

116. S. E. Synderman, L. E. Holt, J. Dancis, E. Roit, A. Boyer, and M. E. Balis, *J. Nutr.* **78:** 57 (1962).

117. D. B. Sprinson, and D. Rittenberg, *J. Biol. Chem.* **180:** 715 (1949).

118. J. M. L. Stephen, *Brit. J. Nutr.* **22:** 153 (1968).

119. J. M. L. Stephen, and J. C. Waterlow, *Lancet* i: 118 (1968).

120. K. Sterling, *J. Clin. Invest.* **30:** 1228 (1951).

121. R. J. C. Stewart and C. R. C. Heard, *Proc. Nutr. Soc.* **18:** 10 (1959).

122. K. L. Stuart, G. Bras, S. J. Patrick, and J. C. Waterlow, *A.M.A. Arch. Intern. Med.* **101:** 67 (1958).

123. M. E. Swendseid, S. G. Tuttle, W. S. Figueroa, D. Mulcare, A. J. Clark, and F. J. Massey, *J. Nutr.* **88:** 239 (1966).

124. A. S. Tavill, A. Craigie, and V. M. Rosenoer, *Clin. Sci.* **34:** 1 (1968).

125. K. Torizuka, K. Hamamoto, K. Koshiyama, K. Iwai, H. Takayama, and T. Miyake, *Metabolism* **12:** 11 (1963).

126. H. C. Trowell, J. N. P. Davies, and R. F. A. Dean, in *Kwashiorkor*. London: Edward Arnold.

127. P. M. Trust, H. Flores, and G. A. O. Alleyne, unpublished observations.

128. A. S. Truswell and J. D. L. Hansen, *S. Afr. Med. J.* **43:** 280 (1969).

129. A. S. Truswell and J. B. Roberts, quoted by Truswell et al. (see 130). (1969).

130. A. S. Truswell, J. D. L. Hansen, C. Watson, and P. Wannenburg, *Amer. J. Clin. Nutr.* **22:** 568 (1969).

131. A. S. Truswell, P. Wannenburg, W. Wittman, and J. D. L. Hansen, *Lancet* i: 1162 (1966).

132. D. P. Tschudy, H. Bacchus, S. Weissman, D. M. Watkin, M. Eubanks, and J. White, *J. Clin. Invest.* **38:** 892 (1959).

133. F. Viteri, M. Behar, G. Arroyave, and N. S. Scrimshaw, in *Mammalian Protein Metabolism*, Vol. II, Chapter 22, H. N. Munro and J. B. Allison, Eds. New York: Academic, (1964).

134. M. Walser and L. J. Bodenlos, *J. Clin. Invest.* **38:** 1617 (1959).

135. J. C. Waterlow, MRC Special Report Series No. 263. H.M.S.O. London (1948).

136. J. C. Waterlow, *Lancet* ii: 1279 (1962).

137. J. C. Waterlow, *Clin. Sci.* **33:** 507 (1967).

138. J. C. Waterlow, *Lancet* ii: 1091 (1968).

139. J. C. Waterlow and T. Weisz, *J. Clin. Invest.* **35:** 346 (1956).

140. J. C. Waterlow and J. M. L. Stephen, *Clin. Sci.* **33:** 489 (1967).

141. J. C. Waterlow and J. M. L. Stephen, *Clin. Sci.* **35:** 287 (1968).

142. J. C. Waterlow, J. Cravioto, and J. M. L. Stephen, *Adv. Protein Chem.* **15:** 131 (1960).

143. G. Weber, R. L. Singhal, and S. K. Srivastara, *Adv. Enzym. Reg.* **3:** 43 (1965).

144. T. Weinstein, G. Dishmon, and M. Heimberg, *Biochem. Pharmacol.* **15:** 851 (1966).

145. L. A. Weller, S. Margen, and D. H. Calloway, *Amer. J. Clin. Nutr.* **22:** 1577 (1969).

146. R. G. Whitehead, *Lancet* i: 250 (1964).

147. R. G. Whitehead, *Lancet* ii: 567 (1965).

148. R. G. Whitehead, *Proc. Nutr. Soc.* **28**: 1 (1969).

149. R. G. Whitehead, and R. F. A. Dean, *Amer. J. Clin. Nutr.* **14**: 313 (1964).

150. R. G. Whitehead, and P. S. E. G. Harland, *Brit. J. Nutr.* **20**: 825.

151. H. G. Windmueller and R. I. Levy, *Circulation* **34**: 239 (1966).

152. H. Wu and S. E. Snyderman, *J. Gen. Physiol.* **34**: 339 (1950).

153. H. Wu and C. W. Bishop, *J. Appl. Physiol.* **14**: 1 (1959).

154. H. Wu and J. Sendroy, *J. Appl. Physiol.* **14**: 6 (1959).

155. H. Wu, J. Sendroy, and C. W. Bishop, *J. Appl. Physiol.* **14**: 11 (1959).

156. T. Yoshida, J. Metcoff, S. Frenk, and C. de la Pena, *Nature* **214**: 525 (1967).

157. T. Yoshida, J. Metcoff, and S. Frenk, *Amer. J. Clin. Nutr.* **21**: 162 (1968).

158. V. R. Young, and N. S. Scrimshaw, *Br. J. Nutr.* **22**: 9 (1968).

159. D. Zilversmit, *Amer. J. Med.* **19**: 832 (1960).

# Index

DA

DEMCO 38-29